WHOLE HEALING

WHOLE HEALING

A STEP-BY-STEP
PROGRAM TO
RECLAIM YOUR
POWER TO HEAL

ELLIOTT S. DACHER, M.D.

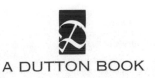

A DUTTON BOOK

DUTTON
Published by the Penguin Group
Penguin Books USA Inc., 375 Hudson Street, New York, New York 10014, U.S.A.
Penguin Books Ltd, 27 Wrights Lane, London W8 5TZ, England
Penguin Books Australia Ltd, Ringwood, Victoria, Australia
Penguin Books Canada Ltd, 10 Alcorn Avenue, Toronto, Ontario, Canada M4V 3B2
Penguin Books (N.Z.) Ltd, 182–190 Wairau Road, Auckland 10, New Zealand

Penguin Books Ltd, Registered Offices:
Harmondsworth, Middlesex, England

First published by Dutton, an imprint of Dutton Signet,
a division of Penguin Books USA Inc.
Distributed in Canada by McClelland & Stewart Inc.

First Printing, May, 1996
10 9 8 7 6 5 4 3 2 1

Excerpt from "Choruses from 'The Rock' " in *Collected Poems 1909–1962* by T. S. Eliot, copyright © 1936 by Harcourt Brace & Company, copyright © 1964, 1963 by T. S. Eliot, reprinted by permission of the publisher.

Dante, *Inferno*, from *The Divine Comedy of Dante Alighieri: Inferno* by Allen Mandelbaum, Translation copyright © 1980 by Allen Mandelbaum. Used by permission of Bantam Books, a division of Bantam Doubleday Dell Publishing Group, Inc.

Mary Oliver, "The Summer Day" from *House of Light* by Mary Oliver. Copyright © 1990 by Mary Oliver. Reprinted by permission of Beacon Press.

W. B. Yeats, "The Second Coming" reprinted with the permission of Simon & Schuster from *The Poems of W. B. Yeats: A New Edition*, edited by Richard J. Finneran. Copyright © 1924 by Macmillan Publishing Company, renewed 1952 by Bertha Georgie Yeats.

René Magritte, "Time Transfixed" © 1996 C. Herscovici, Brussels / Artists Rights Society (ARS), New York

REGISTERED TRADEMARK—MARCA REGISTRADA

LIBRARY OF CONGRESS CATALOGING-IN-PUBLICATION DATA

Dacher, Elliott S.
   Whole healing : a step-by-step program to reclaim your power to heal / Elliott S. Dacher.
      p. cm.
   ISBN 0-525-94155-X
   1. Holistic medicine. 2. Mind and body. 3. Self-care, Health.   I. Title.
R733.D33   1996
615.5—dc20
                                                                    95-47671
                                                                         CIP

Printed in the United States of America
Set in Century Book
Designed by Leonard Telesca

A NOTE TO THE READER
The ideas, procedures, and suggestions contained in this book are not intended as a substitute for consulting with your physician. All matters regarding your health require medical supervision.

*For
the many thousands of
individuals who have passed through
my office and shared their lives with me.
Your pain, suffering, and joy have touched
me deeply and have helped me to grow.
In many ways you have each
contributed to this book, as
you have to my life.*

ACKNOWLEDGMENTS

The transformation of an idea into a book is a communal effort. For this reason it is important for me to name and thank the individuals who contributed to the completion of this project.

I have had the good fortune to work with three editors who, in their own ways, skillfully guided the development of this manuscript. Anita DeVivo contributed her fine editing skills and personal support; John Michel assisted with organizing and presenting the most difficult concepts in this book, always assuring me that sophisticated material, when well written, can be made accessible; and Deirdre Mullane, my editor at Dutton, enthusiastically acquired and then artfully shaped the final manuscript.

Jeanne Fredericks, at a critical moment, assumed the role of my literary agent. Her faith in the material and her persistent and skillful efforts on its behalf found a wonderful home for the book at Dutton. Thanks also to Jody Joy for her able assistance with developing the graphics for this book, and to Leigh-Ann Smith, who carefully and devotedly kept my office going during my absences. Her softness and loyalty are much appreciated.

For as many years as I can remember the Institute of Noetic

Sciences has served as a beacon for those of us who have chosen a more conscious approach to life. I have always felt its presence and support. I would like to give a special thanks to Wink Franklin and Marilyn Schlitz for their ongoing friendship, care, support, and intellectual stimulation. I would also like to convey my appreciation to David Sluyter at the Fetzer Institute, Larry Dossey, and Herb Benson, who have always been present when called upon for assistance and support.

A special thanks to my friends: Adhid Alarif, Luis Albisu, Kathy Eccles, Dawn Ferguson, Peggy Heller, Ann and John McCarty, Brenda Sanchez, Arman and Fera Simone, Eva and Stephen Weinstein, and the group of ten physicians called Metadocs with whom I have met twice yearly for twelve years. Together, we share our lives, ideas, and playfulness. My family, my mom Dora, Kay and Harvey, and my two wonderful daughters Ali and Jessie are always present with their care, support, and love. It is a gift for which there is no proper thank-you.

Finally, it is important for me to give acknowledgment to a group of men and women, including my mom, who in the last decades of their lives have undertaken the study of mind/body healing under the skillful tutelage of Gertrude Friedman in their community of Century Village in West Palm Beach, Florida. The enthusiasm and excitement they have shared with me through their many letters has confirmed my view that health and healing are lifelong endeavors.

CONTENTS

PREFACE

I believe that we each have a destiny and we are responsible for knowing and living this gift with authenticity and love. I discovered years ago that anything less never quite works. At that time, in spite of a carefully and well-conceived set of plans, I found that it was not my destiny to be a physician in the usual sense of that role, or to be satisfied with following a well laid out path of practices and values with the well-known rewards. Although the conventional way would have been an easier one, with more assurance, fewer detours and questions, collegial support that I could count on, and a certain comfort in the doctors' lounge, it has always been wrong for me.

In medical school I spent much of my time working with a fellow medical student establishing a neighborhood health center in a medically impoverished area of Buffalo. Following my internship, I worked for two years as a practicing physician at a model cities health center in a similar area of Boston. Shortly after, much to my surprise, I was invited to become one of the first participants in a Harvard-sponsored effort to establish a primary-care residency program. Although I was appreciative of the opportunity to meet a group of talented individuals and to see scientific medicine at its best, it wasn't quite me. It goes on from there. I was always finding myself in unconventional circumstances, attempting to explore the margins of my profession and to express my own values and beliefs about health and disease.

For many years I tried to assert these values and beliefs within the framework of the medical-care system, but the system and its institutions seemed never quite to follow the wise words of the noted physician Francis Peabody: "The secret of the care of the patient is in caring for the patient." And for me, caring for an individual, as I will discuss shortly, was caring to evoke, in partnership with that individual, the full range of his or her healing capacities. The usual method of "caring for the patient" is limited to a narrow vision of health and healing that diminishes all of us.

I made genuine efforts to work toward my goals within the health-care system, but my soul and spirit kept telling me that it would always be a compromise. The thousands of patients who shared their stories with me, as well as my writing, speaking, personal and professional relationships, and the self-reflection that was forced upon me by a confrontation with my personal wounds, compelled me to accept the fact that I was ill fitted for the role of a conventional physician as it had been taught to me but well fitted to be a very different type of healer. I finally understood that the problem was that the entire institution of medicine has lost its way and no longer remembers its reason for being.

And so I write to use my life experience, an experience that includes 50,000 patient visits, to tell about a new way to approach healing—a way of science, a way of heart, and a way of life. The Whole Healing model, the essential contribution of this book, is the culmination of many years of thought and practice. This model makes use of the capacities of the four healing systems that are built into each of us. When fully used, these capacities provide us with a vast array of healing resources, all under our control. I have used the elements of this model in my life and medical practice, and shared them with many individuals in workshops and conferences. This approach to unlocking our full healing capacities insists that each of us takes back the power to heal that we have inadvertently and inappropriately given to institutions. We have no choice. Institutions cannot heal; only individuals can heal.

As a physician my first concern must be for the welfare of the individual who seeks my help. But I have discovered that any action, whether taken by individuals or professionals, is not only a personal act, but is at the same time a social act, and in the case of healing, a profoundly political act. Consequently, in reclaiming our right to be in charge of an issue as personal as health and healing, we are simultaneously insisting that our cultural institutions support this right, and that the power and authority for health and healing be returned to the individual.

To assume responsibility for our own healing is to confront the system and undermine its authority. In doing so we cause institutions and practitioners to assume a defensive posture. They must guard their investment aggressively while the supposed recipients of the fruits of their science and efforts ask the difficult and probing questions they should be asking. But the institutions and practitioners have a weak defense because of the increasingly apparent limitations of their field, and the increasing fragility and vulnerability of their investment in it.

"The assimilation of a new theory," states Thomas Kuhn, the author of *The Structure of Scientific Revolutions*, "requires the reconstruction of prior theory and the re-evaluation of prior fact, an intrinsically revolutionary process that is seldom completed by a single man and never overnight." So it seems that we are revolutionaries in the midst of an ongoing revolution. We are in this position merely because we need to ask new questions, questions that cannot be answered by the science of our day, and further, we dare to investigate and explore alternative explanations to the issues raised by life and our own natures. And when it comes to the most personal issue of our health, we have, irrespective of the powerful forces that are deeply and perhaps irrevocably invested in the status quo, the right and the obligation to ask questions, to explore possibilities, and to propose alternatives. How else could it be? The practitioners who claim more authority than those they treat must carefully examine the origin of this authority. Those who do will rapidly recognize the inherent fragility of the authority of professional expertise.

There comes a time in any revolution when a vision must be articulated even though to put it in words is invariably to limit it to the concreteness of thought. To fail to articulate a vision, however, is to flounder forever in an endless series of choices, which, regardless of the freedom of unrestricted exploration, denies us the opportunity to fully explore and develop a particular vision. We have diverged enough. There is a time for divergence and a time for convergence. It is now time to converge on a new vision of healing, a new explanatory model, a new worldview. It will not be the last time we do this, but for now we can take the opportunity to move forward, to agree or disagree with this new approach, to refine it progressively, and to test whether this or any other approach best serves the needs of our time. It is through this book, in partnership with the reader, that I hope to explore and practice the medicine of the future—the medicine of Whole Healing.

When I was eight years old I knew that I wanted to be a doctor. My vision was clear, still unaffected by the ways of the world. I remember my initial enthusiasm having, in the words of William Wordsworth, "the glory and the freshness of a dream," but through the years my vision clouded, "The things which I have seen I now can see no more."

I want that vitality back. I want to see again through the wise and clear eyes of adulthood "the glory and freshness of a dream," a dream of a full life—one of caring, commitment, relationship, service, passion, and possibilities. To live this dream is to heal from the inside out. I want this for myself and I want this for all of us. I invite you to join me on this adventure.

—Martha's Vineyard
Summer 1995

INTRODUCTION

A mind that is stretched to a new idea never returns to
its original dimensions.

—Oliver Wendell Holmes

When we get sick we know what to do. We learned the procedure early in life. First we use our common sense, a few days
of rest, or some over-the-counter medications. If we are not
satisfied with our progress, we call for a doctor's appointment.
When we arrive at the office the routine is familiar. Questions
are asked, tests are done, a diagnosis is made, and a treatment
plan is outlined, a plan that usually includes advice, drugs, and
occasionally physical therapy or surgery. These efforts are
usually simple, efficient, and frequently effective. Often, however, modern medicine is less effective with chronic disease,
stress-related illness, fatigue, or the many debilitating symptoms that doctors write off as trivial complaints of "the wor-
ried well"; in these instances we seem to have few options to
choose from. We have learned only one approach to healing.
When it doesn't work we have no place to turn for help.

Physicians are equally frustrated with concerns and complaints that do not fit into the diagnostic categories they were

taught in medical training. Surely if there are no laboratory or X-ray abnormalities, no "physical findings," no specific label or treatment for a problem, it cannot be a "medical" problem. Perhaps it's a psychological problem, a question of burnout from excessive stress, or a chronic disorder predetermined to follow its prescribed downhill course. Physicians, much like their clients, have learned only one approach to disease. If it doesn't work they're stuck.

The past two decades have brought into question the idea that there is only one approach to healing. We have begun to ask ourselves some very important questions: Are there other ways of healing beyond what we know? Do physicians and other health professionals have all the answers? As individuals, can we assist in our own recovery from disease, and further, can we effectively promote our health and well-being? Is health more than the mere absence of disease? The responses to these questions are steadily taking shape, and although they may contain approaches that remind us of healing practices from past eras and other cultures, they are emerging in a form that is unique to our time.

The first response came in the form of the wellness movement, which originated in the 1970s in the teachings and writings of an innovative physician and teacher, Dr. John Travis. Travis challenged us with a simple question. Why, he asked, must we spend our lives moving between only two ways of being—disease and nondisease (the latter state being commonly mistaken for health)? He suggested a third possibility: wellness. Wellness was not a neutral state of no disease, but a positive state of well-being accompanied by feelings of vitality, joyfulness, and energy. Wellness was possible for each of us, as it resulted from our chosen attitudes and lifestyles. The first step, according to Travis, is "a letting go of the archaic belief that disease is something that 'happens' to us at the random direction of forces 'out there.'" This very simple idea of wellness engaged the imaginations of many of us and was the principal driving force in the development of the self-care, fitness, and health-food movements.

Other answers about health came through the popularization of the idea of holism, a term coined by Jan Smuts, a South African prime minister, in his 1926 book *Holism and Evolution*. Holism offered each of us a much larger view of our possibilities than the narrow frame of modern medicine. It offered the perspective that the mind, body, and spirit are at all times interactive and inseparable participants in both the breakdown that leads to disease and the actions that lead to health and well-being. Health and disease were to be found in the unity or disunity of our entire beings, in the manner in which our parts worked together rather than in the dysfunction of one or another piece of our anatomy. We began to realize that we were far more than isolated mechanical bodies helplessly vulnerable to the unexpected occurrence of disease. Further, each of us can call upon the capacities of our minds and bodies to assist with the recovery from disease and the realization of full health. When we learned about holism we discovered that we were not quite as vulnerable, powerless, and innocent as we had thought we were. The idea of holism led us toward its natural result, an exploration of mind/body medicine.

Mind/body medicine opened for each of us the question of how the mind can affect the body, and the related question of how each of us could influence our health through both attitudinal change and specific mind/body practices. We began to explore biofeedback, Yoga, meditation, Tai Chi, imagery, and a host of other approaches to health and healing. Psychoneuroimmunology, an entirely new field of scientific investigation that brings together the study of behavior, the brain, and our natural defense system, the immune system, began to investigate the physiological mechanisms responsible for the mind/body connection. Research in other fields attempted to identify specific personality traits that influence the development of health and disease.

As we explored the mind/body connection, we also began

to question the role of the spirit in issues of health and disease. This led to a rapidly expanding interest in Eastern spiritual practices, and a renewed focus on the healing effects of prayer, love, compassion, service, and relationship. Issues of soul and spirit, however intangible they seemed to our rational minds, touched each of us deeply in places that had long been ignored and forgotten.

The most recent response to our concerns about modern medicine has led to the exploration of alternative and complementary healing practices. These practices, some of which are ancient, such as Chinese and Ayurvedic healing, and others that are more recent, such as homeopathy and chiropractic, are very different from the practices of modern medicine. They do not easily fit into the conventional medical approaches, and we have difficulty deciding which practitioner and practice to try, when and how to use the practice, and of course, how to coordinate them with conventional medicine. The recent establishment of the Office of Alternative Medicine within the framework of the National Institutes of Health is an effort to assist with some of these concerns. That office promotes research that will help to clarify the efficacy and applicability of alternative practices. However, these complicated issues will be with us for a time to come.

Where does all of this leave us? Now, instead of knowing only one way of healing, we are confronted with a diverse set of approaches that have substituted confusion for our previous problem of one-dimensional thinking. What works and what doesn't? When should I use self-care, mind/body practices, conventional practices, and alternative practices? Whom can I trust? Where can I get the reliable information I need? And how does this all fit together? These are the inevitable questions that arise as we question old ways of thinking.

So you may ask, "What is next?" The answer is in this book. For the first time, *Whole Healing* will take us beyond a focus on individual approaches to healing and unfold for the reader what we have all been searching for: an integrated approach to health and healing that will take us past the confusion of the moment toward a clear and concise understanding of integrated healing, an understanding that will fuel our capacity to reclaim ownership of the most personal issue, the issue of health.

We are about to launch an entirely new vision of health and healing. But to do so we must first be willing to learn some basic ground rules. I think of it as somewhat like the investment in learning how to work a computer or run a new software package. We are all familiar with the initial time and effort involved in learning the terminology, reading the manual, and then rereading it, practicing our new skills, and asking others for help. But remember the wonderful feeling of confidence and competence that comes with the mastery of this new information and technology, and the discovery of capacities we never thought possible. All of a sudden we can do more than we could ever do before. We feel empowered, in control of our lives and affairs, and less dependent on others.

It is that way with our health. With a small but consistent effort we can learn how to organize and manage our new options: the power of our minds, bodies, and spirits working together with an expanded array of treatment options. The winner is each of us. What we get is less disease, more choices for recovery and health, and an entirely new vision of health—a vision that offers far more than one way of healing. What we have been missing is an operating system, sort of a control panel like the one that runs our computers and integrates a variety of software packages. Such a system requires an *integrated healing model*. That is the subject of this book.

We begin in Chapter 1 by introducing the details of an integrated healing model, what we call *Whole Healing*. We identify and discuss the four healing systems that are built into the human body. Each of these systems is distinct from the others but only when they are used together is Whole Healing possible. As a complete healing system it provides us with a remarkable capacity for health and healing. As soon as we learn how it works, our ideas about health and healing will undergo a fundamental shift, and what previously seemed like confusion will now appear to be elegant simplicity. We will ask ourselves why we missed something so important, and yet so obvious.

We first learn about our natural self-healing system, the Homeostatic Healing System, how it works, and how we can support and encourage self-healing. We next explore the Treatment Healing System, looking not only at the biomedical approach but at alternative and complementary approaches to healing. We will discover both the value and the inherent liabilities of any treatment system. Then our journey into the Mind/Body Healing System unveils for us some new and important facts. We will find that mind/body healing is not exclusively about self-regulation, practices that manipulate the body through the use of the mind, but rather about the full development of our minds, a process that leads to both psychological and physiological health. Finally, we explore the Spiritual Healing System, which when activated has an extraordinary capacity to reorganize our psychology and physiology in a direction that assists with recovery and insures health.

We will also learn how to recognize the qualities of health, qualities that emerge as we activate the Mind/Body Healing System. Although we know a great deal about the signs and symptoms of disease, few have given any attention to the signs and symptoms of health. To know what health looks like is to be able to orient ourselves in the right direction. I'll discuss seven qualities of health as gleaned from my experience with thousands of patients and my survey of the few noted experts who have asked the important but usually overlooked question, What are the "signs and symptoms" of health?

As we continue on our journey, we will discover that even though biomedicine is highly technical, we now have the capacity to orchestrate our personal health. This does not require a technical expertise, but rather an expertise in managing our health. We will learn about accessing reliable information, choosing and "working" a specific healing system, investigating different healing practices, and applying what we have learned to the circumstances of our lives.

Finally, we will conclude our exploration by considering our major resource for health: ourselves. We will discover that no belief system, expert, or institution can do for us what we can and must do for ourselves, an effort that is made possible only through an integrated approach to Whole Healing.

I would like to offer you some suggestions for maximizing what you can learn from this book. Read a chapter at a time, and if necessary, reread it. Practice the exercises, and carefully and critically consider the issues raised in each chapter. Work with them in your mind, discuss them with your friends, and identify how they apply to your life. You are not alone. You are joining me and others as cocreators of a new healing system. We all started with one way of healing, and now we are discovering that more is possible. Take your time and enjoy the process.

WHOLE HEALING

The real voyage of discovery rests not in seeking
new landscapes, but in having new eyes.
—Marcel Proust

I met Marie on a long cross-country flight. She was returning to her home in California after a business trip. We spoke about oceans and beaches, and I told her how much I was looking forward to a few days of long walks by the sea. After a heavy sigh she said, "I've lived near the beach for the past year and I haven't been able to take one walk." Although she didn't know I was a physician, she continued to speak with some intensity: "I've had asthma for two years, and now it is so severe that I have to stay indoors as much as possible." She continued, "I'm too young to stop doing all the things I love to do." As I listened, I wondered whether physicians have a subtle way of attracting those who are ill, or whether it was my smile of encouragement that invited her disclosures. Either way, I put my work aside to listen.

In the past two years she had seen numerous physicians, had undergone complete allergy testing, and had taken the usual prescribed medicines. Despite these efforts her symptoms were getting worse. "It's the pollen," she said. "I know it's the pollen." She continued with this thought in a rather persistent way even though I pointed out to her that she had lived in the same area for many years without any previous problem with asthma. I took another tack, asking "Was there something that happened in your life before the asthma began?" A bit set back by what seemed to be an irrelevant question, she responded, "No, nothing."

Because I have heard so many similar stories, I pressed on with some ambivalence (after all I was taking an airplane flight, not conducting an office visit). "Think carefully," I told her, then asked again, "Did anything unusual happen in your life?" After a pause she spoke. "Well, now that I think about it my mother died around the time I got my first attack."

"What happened?" I asked. She responded, "I've never been close to my mother, but on the day she died she had complained of some chest pain. She had similar pains many times before, but I told her I would come over. She insisted that it wasn't necessary, but I knew I should have gone. She died that night, and I feel guilty."

Noticing her sadness, I asked, "What have you done about the guilt, and sadness, and anger?" "What do you mean?" she answered. "Well," I asked, "when did the asthma start?" "About a month later," she responded, not making the connection between the events in her life and her disease.

As we talked it became clear. Marie had come to believe that disease generally has a single cause, one that is usually outside of ourselves. In her case it was pollen. A single cause calls for a magic bullet, which for us means drugs. And even though all her efforts at such treatment had failed to heal her asthma, she persisted in using that treatment.

Through their experience, physicians learn that there is a time to join an individual compassionately in his or her pain and suffering, and a time to confront. With only an hour left on the flight I realized that I would have to take the path of confrontation. I let her know that I was a doctor, and stated my view as clearly as possible. "Disease is not caused by one external agent," I said, "nor is it ever isolated to one part of ourselves. Disease results from the combination of many issues that lead to a disunity in our mind and body. Disease is a disorder of our whole being. Your asthma," I stated, "can be fully healed."

I went on to say that healing would require her to understand the full web of circumstances, inner and outer, that resulted in the disunity of mind and body that she called asthma. I told her that she could learn about and apply her own built-in capacities for healing, moving from her present partial approach to healing to one of Whole Healing. I also assured her that if she chose to engage her disease in this way then she would walk on the beaches again. She listened intently, yet skeptically, and asked me where to begin. I told her that I would find someone in her area who could help her with the first steps toward Whole Healing. Within a few days I called her to fulfill my promise.

For Marie, the problem was a severely limited understanding of her disease and her own healing capacities. For others who are exploring for the first time the rich diversity of healing approaches that are now increasingly available, the problem is very different. Consider the following.

Several months ago I received a telephone call from Ann, a thirty-two-year-old woman in considerable emotional distress. Although we had never met before, her story came quickly as she sought my advice and assistance. Four months previously she had been diagnosed with a localized, surgically curable, cancer of the cervix. For the next month she reflected on her options and then decided to forgo surgery. Instead, she traveled to a Mexican clinic to try an alternative therapy. After three weeks of that therapy she was advised to return home and undergo the previously recommended surgery. She did so. At the time of surgery the surgeon explored the cancer and found that it had progressed. What had been an easily curable cancer had now advanced. Four months before, this woman could anticipate many more years. Her potential now for a long and full life were dramatically changed. In her call to me she was struggling to make sense of the situation.

In Marie's situation the problem was a lack of information. In Ann's circumstance there were newly discovered alternative practices, a burgeoning number of options for healing, and plenty of information, but no way to sort through them and organize them for her benefit. These two people are typical of many people who seek medical help. Most do not have an understanding of their capacity for healing themselves, and even if they do, they have a lot of information but no effective way to use it. So the absence of information is only part of the problem. How to use information, particularly when it is plentiful, is the second part of the problem.

Ironically, we are living in a time when we are no longer dependent on a single health-care system and its particular perspectives. We are now discovering multiple unrelated health-care systems such as Ayurveda, Chinese medicine, and homeopathy; each has its own logic, approach, and treatment options, each is rapidly expanding our information and capacities for healing. Yet this sudden embarrassment of riches has resulted in a fragmented approach to healing. Some people are unaware of these new opportunities, and others who are aware make decisions based on pieces of information, pieces that too often are taken out of context and can therefore be more misleading than helpful. The problem is simply this: At a time when our world is changing and our possibilities are expanding, we have not yet developed a way to find the best and most direct route to health and healing.

This problem has developed in part because we are living at a time when old structures and ways of thinking are coming apart and new ideas are being formulated. This shift in our way of thinking can be most dramatically seen in the reshaping of our ideas about health and healing. We are changing from a mechanical view of the mind and body, one that examines and repairs one cog, one spring, and one flywheel at a time, to one that is dynamic and holistic. This shift has given rise to confusion and, at times, false hopes, but it has also given rise to a fundamentally new set of opportunities. Yet with all the changes that are occurring, several clear facts emerge:

• We no longer believe that there is a single cause for each illness. We now recognize that disease, like health, is the result of a web of circumstances that involve our mind, body, spirit, and environment.

• We no longer believe that there is only one way to heal. We now recognize that no singular approach, practice, or treatment has all the answers.

• We no longer believe that the power to heal is exclusively contained in external agents or treatments. We now recognize the wealth of healing capacities that are built into our minds, bodies, and spirits.

• We no longer believe that health professionals have all the answers to our questions about health and disease. We now recognize that there are answers we must seek ourselves.

A new vision of healing cannot be found through any one healing practice or a combination of them. Nor can it be found by shifting our focus from the body to the mind, or from one practitioner to another. Healing does not evolve from the proper functioning of pieces and parts, from the exclusive influence of either the mind or body, or from one system of belief or another. It emerges from our entire experience, which gives us access to all the possibilities for both inner and outer healing. The task becomes a process of exploring and bringing into our lives a fundamentally new and comprehensive approach to healing, an approach that I call *Whole Healing*.

SOLVING THE PROBLEM

As we move along the path toward Whole Healing, here is what we need: first, an understanding of the Whole-Healing process and a new vision of what it means to be healthy; second, the capacity to choose intelligently among the extensive menu of practices and approaches—conventional, alternative, mind/body, and spiritual; and third, an understanding of how these approaches work together. These three essential elements of a complete healing program were the missing ingredients in Marie's and Ann's quests for healing.

To facilitate these steps we need a way to consolidate the current array of healing practices into a coherent process, one that serves our needs rather than adding conflict and confusion. We must answer these questions: How do we expand our knowledge and understanding of our full healing capacities? How do we create order and coherence out of diversity? How do we bring together what appear to be separate aspects of healing into a natural whole that can serve our day-to-day health concerns while promoting long-term health? These are the questions that Marie and Ann, unknowingly, were beginning to ask for each of us. Their dilemmas reflected the larger concerns that we are all now confronting. The answers to these questions will force us to break through the limitations of a partial and inadequate approach to healing.

I'd like to propose a model that achieves that consolidation by considering the full range of healing already available to us, the four distinct healing systems that we can identify as part of our personal experience. Each of these systems has its own frame of reference, operating principles, characteristics, practitioners, practices, and research methodologies. I call the four systems Homeostasis, Treatment, Mind/Body, and Spiritual. At any one time, most of us are using one or two of these systems. That is what we are taught and what we are accustomed to. Used individually, these systems are limited and partial approaches to healing. Taken together, they form a Whole Healing System with a flexibility, adaptability, and comprehensiveness that cannot be accounted for by the mere sum of the individual components.

The figure below illustrates the natural nesting of the four individual systems to form a single whole. In the pages that follow we will examine each of the systems separately, but it is important to remember that in life they always operate as a unity, as one system. Living systems do not exist as parts; it is only our capacity for abstraction that makes it seem this way. And although the chapters in this book on the individual healing systems can each stand alone as descriptions of separate and distinct healing paths, human life, as we know it, is dependent on the presence and interaction of *all* of these four systems.

THE HEALTH CONTINUUM

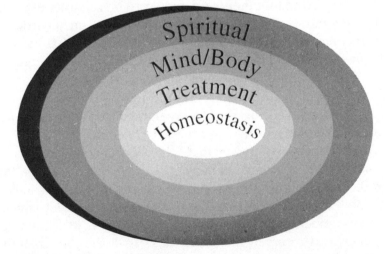

The Whole Healing System is composed of four separate and unique healing systems. Each system builds upon the other systems by adding new capacities and resources. In our lives, the entire system works as one, providing us with a remarkable capacity for self-healing.

As we consider each of the systems we will see how they share six basic characteristics, and how these typical characteristics of healing come together in a unique way in each of the four systems. Each draws upon a different aspect of consciousness, operates through a unique mechanism and process, and applies its resources to achieving a particular aspect of health. As we add one system to the others we will notice an expansion of consciousness, an increasing number of available resources for healing, and an enlarging sense of what it means to be healthy. We will discover that health is many things: a well-functioning mind and body, the capacity to recover from disease, the development of personal autonomy, and the progressive achievement of wholeness.

In building a new model of health we must also remember that it is *person centered*. We may automatically think that our intention is to build a better health-care system. This is not our goal. Systems cannot heal us. A person-centered healing model begins with a focus on our innate healing capacities, in the form of the four healing systems. Think of them as the hub of a wheel. They are the central focus and support of the wheel. At times we may reach out to the periphery to call upon other healing resources, professionals, practices, or treatments, to complement our built-in capacities. But these resources, when effectively used, can only assist us when they support rather than attempt to substitute for our natural healing systems. Health-care systems assume that health can be designed and delivered to us through some generic social formula. Whole Healing knows that health is a diverse, unique, and highly personal experience.

THE HOMEOSTATIC HEALING SYSTEM

In 1929 Walter Cannon, the famed physician-physiologist, described the most primary and basic healing system available to us: the homeostatic system. This inborn system of internal physiological checks and balances, which evolved over the millennia of human development, makes it possible for us to respond automatically to internal states of disequilibrium with immediate, reflexlike physiological corrections. As a result, body temperature, fluid and mineral balance, and other automatic activities are kept in balance at all times. In this way homeostatic healing contributes to our health by maintaining a constant internal environment—a necessity for life.

HOMEOSTASIS

Consciousness	Instinctual
Mechanism	Autoregulation
Process	Checks and Balances
Focus	Disequilibrium
Resources	Feedback Loops
Health	Steady State

The Homeostatic Healing System, which is built in at birth, is our most primary healing system. It operates through the automatic activation of an array of internal checks and balances that assure that the body functions in a manner that can sustain life. Each draws upon a different aspect of consciousness, operates through a unique mechanism and process, and applies its resources to achieving a particular aspect of health.

The Homeostatic Healing System developed into its present form through a progressive accumulation of checks and balances designed to respond to the disruptive effects of internal and external stresses on our physiology, stresses that would tend to shift our system toward imbalance. However, because it takes approximately 1 million years to accomplish a 5 percent sustained change in the human biological system, our homeostatic system is far more suited to the life of our ancient ancestors than it is to the more recent and dramatic changes in lifestyle and environment that characterize urban life. As a result, the homeostatic system, a relatively fixed and unchanging system, is often poorly adapted to the lifestyles, practices, and environments of our day-to-day lives: our nutritional choices, exercise patterns, physical environments, and, above all, our stress levels. This mismatch of our inherited natural protective mechanisms to the realities of a twentieth-century lifestyle have resulted in significant limitations and deficiencies in the effectiveness of this system.

For example, consider the human stress response that evolved as a quick on-and-off reaction to the abrupt appearance of physical danger. In modern times, lions no longer appear suddenly in the bush, causing a heightened sense of alarm, only to disappear shortly thereafter. Our modern "lions" take the form of worries, fears, and anxieties, which constantly activate the stress response. Worse, unlike our ancient ancestors, through conscious intervention we can block or avoid the natural response, which is to escape from or avoid stressful and dangerous situations. For intellectual reasons, we often choose to remain in stressful circumstances so that our stress response is, ironically, activated. When this happens, the normal protective response, which once insured survival, is unable to respond effectively to the new realities of our lives, and the result is the development of acute and chronic stress-related disease. What once insured the survival of life now can threaten our survival.

It is important that we learn to understand and use each of the healing systems in order to maximize what each has to offer. With the Homeostatic Healing System we can best support and enhance its effectiveness by providing the environment, nutrition, and physical activity that most approximates the circumstances under which it developed. To a large extent these activities fall under the label of "prevention." In a sense, we are attempting to prevent a malfunction of this system by giving it what it needs. Perpetual mental stress, high fat intake, processed foods, and a sedentary lifestyle are creations of urban life that do not support homeostasis.

But there is more to maintaining the homeostatic system than these physical requirements. We cannot overlook the fact that our ancestors spent their lifetimes with the same 100 to 150 people, had a cosmology that brought meaning and wonder to their existence, and experienced lives that were well integrated into the natural patterns and cycles of nature. I am not suggesting a return to such times; this would be neither possible nor preferable. But when we understand the circumstances under which the homeostatic system developed, we can appreciate the value of inner peace, natural foods, exercise, relationships, and a vital spirit. In each case we close the gap between our inherited balancing mechanisms and our current lifestyles, nurturing our natural protective mechanisms. In a sense, by learning to respect the needs of our bodies, we learn to respect what has been given to us and to align ourselves better with nature, an action that has implications well beyond the boundaries of our personal world.

Nature's extreme way of reminding and forcing us to comply with the basic needs of this system takes the form of sickness. Our natural protective mechanisms fail, our bodies force us to slow down, rest, reach out to others, and reconsider our lifestyles. When we persist in perpetuating attitudes and lifestyles that are inconsistent with our natural needs, ignoring the messages from our bodies, these personal choices can influence the transformation of acute illness into chronic degenerative illness, disability, and premature death. There is always a physical and psychological price for disregarding our nature. Health, growth, and fulfillment occur in partnership with our nature, not in resistance to it.

To remedy the deficiencies of a fixed and too often maladaptive Homeostatic Healing System, we have developed "treatment" models whose purpose is to step in and restore normal function when homeostasis has failed. Treatment practices, conventional and alternative, increasingly draw upon man-made interventions, which, unlike our automatic protective mechanisms, are flexible and can respond to changing conditions. To an extent we can say that our capacity to design treatment systems that augment nature's mechanisms reflects our progress as humans. One can also say it is an indication of how far, for better or for worse, we have removed ourselves from nature.

THE TREATMENT HEALING SYSTEM

Treatment, in its various forms, is the dominant model of healing in Western culture. The figure below illustrates the major characteristics of this system. It is activated by our reaction to the signs and symptoms of illness, and works toward repairing abnormalities through the use of external resources such as drugs and surgery. As we shall discuss in more detail in the next chapter, practitioners first seek to establish the singular cause of the problem, and then apply their resources to the goal of restoring normal function. At one time or another each of us will use the resources of the treatment system to address the inevitable adversities of living.

To treat is to apply a process to a problem with the intention of resolving it. In the case of biomedical treatment the process usually consists of the use of external agents such as drugs, surgery, or physical therapy. Other forms of treatment may come in the form of vitamins and other supplements, biofeedback, relaxation techniques, body work, energy work, chiropractic, acupuncture, and a host of other practices. We activate treatment when we seek assistance from a health-care practitioner as a reaction to the appearance of a symptom, or the presence of overt disease, an indication of the breakdown of the Homeostatic Healing System. The initial complaint is routinely followed by the requisite testing, the establishment of a diagnosis, and the prescription of therapy according to the particular practice, a therapy that is usually directed at a specific body part. Decisions are made by the health professional, and treatment is exclusively dictated by the type of disease. Treatment is generally tailored to the *disease* rather than to the unique characteristics and needs of the *individual* within whom the disorder expresses itself.

In general, treatment approaches are developed from fields of study that seek to understand the cause of the symptom and disease by narrowing in on a single body system, organ, cell, or, in the case of biomedicine, on biochemistry. The idea that a malfunction of the body can always be attributed to a specific abnormality localized at the biochemical, cellular, tissue, or organ level is called reductionism. This single-cause theory implies that the human body is an organized collection of parts that generally function independently of environmental, psychosocial, and spiritual influences. The idea is to find the singular abnormality and then to discover the "magic bullet" or practice that will cure it. The goal is to repair the abnormality and to reestablish health, which, in the treatment system, is defined as the restoration of normal function.

TREATMENT

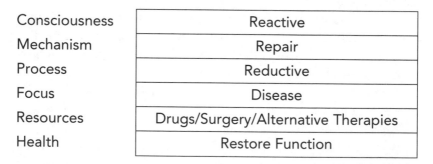

Consciousness	Reactive
Mechanism	Repair
Process	Reductive
Focus	Disease
Resources	Drugs/Surgery/Alternative Therapies
Health	Restore Function

The Treatment Healing System relies upon the use of external agents, treatments, and practices, usually provided by a professional, for the purpose of repairing abnormalities and restoring normal function. There are many different approaches to treatment, each differing in theory and practice.

This method is similar to the way we approach a car or machine: We first look the whole thing over and then narrow in on the broken part. But what works for machines doesn't work for people. In the treatment approach, the subjective and personal experience of an individual is considered "noise" and is ignored. Too often it is disregarded by the individual as well as the practitioner, both of whom learned this through culture and formal education. Marie's experience with asthma is a typical example. Asthma is exclusively seen as a disorder of the breathing tubes, which causes them to go into spasm inappropriately, interrupting the flow of air to the lungs. This disorder is seen a result of a biochemical instability that causes an excessive reactivity of the airways, particularly to airborne pollens and other such substances. The treatment is to diminish this reactivity with a variety of medications. The advice given to physicians by the famed internist Sir William Osler is instructive: He said, "It is better to know the person that has the disease, than the disease that has the person." As we can see in Marie's situation it would have greatly contributed to her healing to have "known the patient who has the disease" as well as "the disease that has the patient." This wisdom applies to Marie and her health professionals, both of whom knew much about asthma and its treatments but little about Marie.

Because Western medicine is the most frequently used form of treatment, let's use it as an example. Biomedicine has achieved its greatest success within very specific areas: anesthesia, surgery, immunization, and the antibiotic treatment of bacterial infections. Its expanding base of scientific knowledge has provided us with both an extensive, although narrowly focused, understanding of disease and extraordinary diagnostic and therapeutic strategies. New forms of treatment, improved public health, and increasing levels of affluence have resulted in an extension of the average life span from forty years at the onset of this century to a current seventy-five years.

However, the success of biomedicine has also exposed its severe limitations. Those successful treatments, public-health measures, rising levels of affluence, and urban lifestyles that are a consequence of the industrial revolution have also resulted in a dramatic shift in the kinds of illness we suffer from. Instead of epidemics of acute infectious disease, we now have epidemics of chronic, often stress-related, degenerative diseases whose causes are largely a result of harmful environments, changing lifestyles, personal attitudes, unhealthy relationships, and unresolved conflict. Biomedicine is well equipped to diagnose and treat degenerative diseases, but its therapies rarely result in cure because in general treatment fails to address the primary sources of these diseases, the unique web of circumstances within an individual's life that results in a disunity of mind, body, and spirit.

Much the same can be said about other treatments. It is currently fashionable to call many interventions and techniques holistic, suggesting that they aim at something beyond the goal of treatment. But the facts tell a different story. However well intentioned a practitioner may be, a practice strategy that involves one person (usually considered the expert) doing something to someone else most often falls under the treatment system as we know it. Although the intellectual intention of a practitioner and a client may lean toward holism, the practice and its impact may be quite different. The effort, regardless of the rhetoric, is usually directed toward repair and restoration of function, leaving the individual without further empowerment or enhanced personal skills and resources.

As with the homeostatic system, an understanding of the treatment system, its assets and limitations, demonstrates the need for an enhanced approach to healing. Exclusive use of a treatment system, by its very definition, is incapable of *meaningfully* including psychological and social aspects of our lives. These factors cannot be reduced to the level of biochemistry, cells, tissues, or organ systems without disregarding their meaning and significance to us. And while many practitioners are beginning to combine treatment with mind/body and spiritual approaches, this is still the exception, and many find it difficult to shift from being an "expert" in a particular practice to a shared practitioner-client relationship, a partnership that is an essential requirement of a broader-based approach to healing.

THE MIND/BODY HEALING SYSTEM

As we leave homeostasis and treatment to consider mind/body and spiritual healing we move from an automatic system that is inborn and a treatment system that is culturally imposed from without to systems of healing that rely on our consciousness and intention. Unlike the first two systems, mind/body and spiritual healing offer us the capacity for self-regulation and self-exploration, and in doing so give us the opportunity for a more direct and personal involvement in our health.

Unlike the physical context of the homeostatic and treatment systems, the Mind/Body and Spiritual Healing Systems evoke a very different view of the human condition. These systems call upon the capacities and qualities that characterize human life: consciousness, intention, will, creativity, faith, love, and compassion. In these systems we deal less with parts and increasingly focus on the wholes. The Mind/Body and Spiritual Healing Systems operate through "downward" causation, the process by which higher levels of human organization, the mind and spirit, effect changes in cells, tissues, and organ systems by reorganizing the whole. This is in contrast to the idea of "upward causation," with the parts determining the status of the whole. (I will cover these concepts more fully in the next chapter.) Both of these ideas of causation are valid, and it is important that a comprehensive healing system consider and incorporate both.

The Mind/Body Healing System relies on personal responsibility and self-motivated effort. It requires the development and use of personal skills and capacities—physical, psychological, and psychosocial—that can help us connect mind, body, and spirit, and the development of the capacity for self-regulation. In contrast to homeostasis, which operates automatically, and the various forms of treatment, which are applied in response to the appearance of disease, mind/body healing is proactive and intentional. Its focus is on personal attitudes and lifestyles, and the skills that are necessary for healthy relationships, conflict resolution, and personal growth and development, the critical components of a health-promotion program.

MIND/BODY HEALING

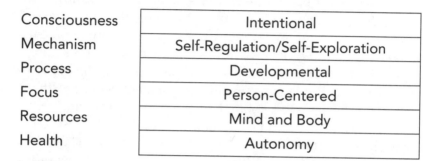

Consciousness	Intentional
Mechanism	Self-Regulation/Self-Exploration
Process	Developmental
Focus	Person-Centered
Resources	Mind and Body
Health	Autonomy

The Mind/Body Healing system is activated through personal choice and initiative. The expansion of consciousness, access to a more comprehensive self-understanding, and the development of new skills and resources lead to a progressive capacity for self-regulation.

The full potential of this system is developed over time as a result of our choices and our efforts. It is neither automatic, like the homeostatic system, nor culturally imposed, like the treatment system. We have a choice, to develop its potential or not. It is a person-centered system rather than a disease-centered one. Mind/body healing is concerned with psychological development, personal transformation, and mastery, to the extent possible, over the activities of the mind and body.

This aspect of healing bases its scientific legitimacy on the emerging research in the field of psychoneuroimmunology. The discovery that the interconnectedness of our thoughts, feelings, images, and biochemistry is mediated through a mobile neuropeptide messenger system, a series of natural chemicals that transfer information between the mind and body, has provided us with an understanding of the biochemical pathways that link the mind and the body. To the extent that our emotions and chemistry are linked, how we develop psychologically influences the physiology of our bodies. Research is now demonstrating the relationship between certain feeling states, attitudes, and perspectives and their effect on our biochemistry, for example, how feelings can suppress the immune system. Further, we are becoming increasingly aware, as we'll see later, of how our attitudes and actions can enhance our resistance to the detrimental effects of excessive stress. In short, we are learning how to *evoke health*.

The change in focus from diagnostic categories to issues of personal attitudes, lifestyles, and psychological development alters the relationship of the health practitioner to his patient. This interaction becomes more of a partnership, in contrast to the hierarchical relationship that characterizes the treatment system. The focus is long-term, and treatment, which can more accurately be termed "self-regulation," is more internal than external. The intent of the mind/body system is more educational than therapeutic, and a health practitioner serves more as an educator and coach. The skills required are very different from those taught in conventional practitioner training programs. They include expanded psychological skills, communication skills, and an awareness of the practices that serve as resources for this aspect of healing. It is at this level of healing that we most profoundly see the shift from outer aids to inner resources.

To maximize the effectiveness of the homeostatic healing system we need only to adhere to some basic health practices. In the case of the treatment system we need only comply with the directions of the practitioner. When it comes to mind/body healing, however, we need some instruction. The first part of the mind/body curriculum is learning a variety of practices that develop the skills, resources, and capacities for self-regulation. There are many to choose from including: meditation, Yoga, breathing techniques, Tai Chi, Aikido, imagery, biofeedback, art, dance, writing, and journaling. Each of these practices, and many others, is something we can do for ourselves in contrast to something that is done *to* us. We become our own healers, applying intention, will, commitment, and persistence to our efforts to develop our healing system fully. In this manner we discover that when we pay attention to our lives, many of our most potent sources of healing can be found in the routine activities of our day-to-day lives.

The second aspect of mind/body healing is learning how to more deeply observe and understand our individual lives. In particular, we can learn new ways of approaching health and disease, relationships, communication, conflict, and career choices. The expansion of self-knowledge will provide us with an understanding of the workings of the mind, an expansion of consciousness, and a deeper and richer sense of a very different self. There are many techniques that offer help in the expansion of self-understanding. These include meditation, psychotherapy, twelve-step programs, self-help groups, reading, seminars, and, of most importance, an ongoing process of self-inquiry.

Just as the focus of mind/body healing differs from that of homeostasis and treatment, their goals also differ. Homeostasis defines health as the maintenance of a steady state, and treatment aims at restoring normal function. Mind/body healing incorporates these aspects of health, but extends them to include the expansion of consciousness and self-knowledge, and the acquisition of new skills and resources, an adventure that continues throughout a lifetime. As we shall see in the following chapters, at this level our definition of health slowly shifts from preoccupation with sporadic episodes of illness toward a concern with the more creative and personal act of designing a healthy life.

As with the homeostatic and treatment systems, the defining focus of the Mind/Body Healing System, self-awareness and psychological development, accounts for its contributions as well as its limitations. This system approaches but fails to fully consider the spiritual aspects of human experience that transcend and extend the boundaries of personal development. To convey a holistic and intuitive understanding of the living experience that in itself is healing, the Spiritual Healing System comes into play.

THE SPIRITUAL HEALING SYSTEM

Although the spiritual experience is singular in nature, there are many paths to it and different names for it. It can arise quite suddenly, through the experience of prayer, devotion, love, compassion, meditation, music, dance, art, and nature. It may last a few precious brief moments, or, at times, for longer periods. It can also evolve slowly over a lifetime of study, practice, growth, and development. In the latter instance, it is as if small islands of understanding expand and coalesce over many years to provide a more comprehensive awareness and understanding of the whole of life.

The spiritual perspective is a way of understanding life that provides meaning to our day-to-day experiences and the larger issues of living and dying. Spirituality sees wholes rather than parts, and patterns rather than details. When we are guided by this perspective, life seems to make sense, everything is in its place, and we feel balanced and connected. This deeper sense

SPIRITUAL HEALING

Consciousness	Intuitive
Mechanism	Integration
Process	Unifying
Focus	Myth/Symbol
Resources	Consciousness
Health	Wholeness

The Spiritual Healing System is activated when we experience a sense of wholeness. This experience, through its profound effect on our attitudes and perspectives, is healing to the mind and body. It can be activated spontaneously for brief moments, or developed through a progressive expansion of consciousness.

of self and nature is satisfying to the soul and spirit. It can have profound effects on personal attitudes, values, relationships, and unresolved conflicts, and as a consequence it can influence biochemistry and physiology. I call these effects on the mind and body spiritual healing.

Unlike the preceding healing systems, spiritual healing results from a way of *being* rather than *doing*. While mind/body healing results in an increasing sense of peace and understanding, spiritual healing conveys wisdom and a persistent sense of oneness with life. In its emphasis on wholeness, spiritual healing relies on intuitive knowledge, an often unused aspect of our consciousness. It operates by conveying to us a unifying and integrated vision of life, and a sense of meaning, purpose, and coherence. The spiritual experience cannot be well characterized through the limitations of descriptive prose. It is best communicated through symbols, art, poetry, sacred spaces, religion, and myth.

As we consider the Spiritual Healing System it is necessary to point out that healing can be, and has been, approached from two directions. Throughout much of Western history, people relied on faith and spirit as the predominant focus of healing. Individual development, what we have termed mind/body healing, was inconsequential, if not heretical. Through the exclusive and disciplined practice of faith, often in the form of organized religion, day-to-day life was maintained in a state of peace and balance. This is not to suggest that faith in itself resolved and healed all disease, but rather that it provided a continuity and transcendent meaning to life that allowed for an inner peace and balance, mental and physical. But ours is not such a time, and the vast majority of us will find it necessary to discover the transcendent through the exploration and progressive understanding of our day-to-day lives, our relationships, conflicts, and life transitions. For us the path to Whole Healing is not downward from, what would seem to us, an uninformed faith, but rather through the process of individuation and personal transformation, a process that is uniquely Western and modern in character.

There is no "better" or "worse" here, merely our historical circumstance, one from which we cannot escape.

USING THE HEALTH CONTINUUM

As we explore the four healing systems as a single, fully integrated model, we can discern qualities that are related not to the individual healing systems but to the healing system as an indivisible whole. The result is somewhat like the relationship of individual notes to the melody found in a musical composition. The notes are the elements of the music, yet the music is much more than just notes. The rhythm, the arrangement of the notes, and the spaces between them give the work as a whole a certain context, movement, significance, and meaning. We find in the musical composition a dynamism and vitality that is not a property of the notes by themselves, but only emerges through their organized interaction.

And so it is with the Whole Healing System. Each of the individual systems taken alone is static, stationary, and devoid of the dynamism of life. But if we take them together we find a fully integrated, moving, flexible, adaptive, and organic process. It is all *one* carefully orchestrated process that comes alive only as we consider the whole.

It has been often said that there are no colleges that teach us about healing, or for that matter, about life. We are left either to rely on others or to do the best we can through self-study and trial and error. But the new model of Whole Healing that we've been exploring can serve as a guide to the development of our healing powers. Movement from one system to the next is marked by an initiation. We are initiated into homeostasis through our birth, into treatment through our family and culture, and into mind/body and spiritual healing through the major breakdowns and setbacks of our lives, of which disease is certainly one. Instead of traveling the road without a map, we now have one. The Whole Healing model is a guide to the

WHOLE HEALING

	Homeostasis	Treatment	Mind/Body	Spiritual
Consciousness	Instinctual	Reactive	Intentional	Intuitive
Mechanism	Autoregulation	Repair	Self-Regulation/Self-Exploration	Integration
Process	Checks & Balances	Reductive	Developmental	Unifying
Focus	Disequilibrium	Disease	Person-Centered	Myth/Symbol
Resources	Feedback Loops	Drugs/Surgery Alternative Therapies	Mind/Body	Consciousness
Health	Steady State	Restore Function	Autonomy	Wholeness

The Whole Healing model, when looked at in its entirety, is a guide to the progressive development of consciousness, the expansion of personal resources and capacities, the unfolding of a larger vision of health, the attainment of wholeness, and, of course, Whole Healing.

development of our healing capacities, our consciousness, and our evolving sense of what it means to be healthy.

In my own life and in my work with clients I frequently refer to this model and ask the questions, Where am I (or where is my client) on the developmental continuum? What is called for at this stage of life? What aspect(s) of healing are essential at this time? Consider the following example.

Richard, a forty-five-year-old lawyer, comes to my office with the symptoms of atherosclerotic heart disease. His age and the intensity and severity of this particular illness indicate the need to consider, at a minimum, the Treatment and Mind/Body Healing Systems. Further inquiry, which may continue over weeks, will clarify whether Richard is willing to and capable of viewing his disease within the framework of a spiritual perspective, a perspective that is both appropriate and essential for his age. Stated another way, is he ready to "use" his disease as a challenge to transform his life, to take some risks and explore new possibilities? First, I would discuss with him and then initiate appropriate steps toward treatment, diagnosis, and therapy. Next we would examine the context of his illness, the web of circumstances, attitudes, and lifestyles that has brought him to this point in his life. Finally, if it is acceptable to him, we would begin a dialogue together in which we would seek a larger understanding of the meaning, purpose, significance, and implications of this disease for his life.

In this case a Whole Healing plan includes a mixture of approaches: the use of appropriate diagnostic and therapeutic interventions (the treatment system), the introduction of attitudinal and lifestyle changes in the areas of stress management, nutrition, exercise, conflict resolution, and insight-based psychological counseling (the mind/body system), and an ongoing consideration of the impact of this illness on previously held values, beliefs, and priorities (the spiritual system). The goal is to use this disease as a doorway into a more considered and expanded life—one that serves to remedy the problem at hand, to reverse the personal factors that have contributed to the development of the illness, and to enhance the overall quality of life.

Consider again the case of Ann, whom we saw earlier in this chapter. How would I have worked with her if I had met her at the time of diagnosis? To begin with, I would have strongly recommended that she immediately proceed with the surgical treatment of the tumor, a use of the treatment system that would likely have cured the cancer. Then I would have quickly introduced her to a variety of mind/body practices, such as meditation and imagery, that could have helped her in preparing for surgery and assisted her during the recovery period. Once the immediate issues were handled, I would have spent time discussing with her how, by examining her attitudes and lifestyle—issues of food, exercise, and stress—she could possibly influence the risk of a second cancer (individuals with cancer are at an increased risk of a second cancer). Finally, we would begin the most important part of our conversation, exploring the significance of this life-threatening disease, what it can teach her about her life, her directions, and her priorities. Together we would seek to find a meaning to this phase of her life, a meaning to help transform the next part of her life, a path to renewal and wholeness. The Whole Healing of a disease of this severity requires the use of the entire healing system. The result is not only the elimination of the illness, but the promotion of health and the revitalization and redirection of life.

As we begin to understand the implications of Whole Healing we will naturally loosen our exclusive reliance on practitioners. It will become quite evident that the capacity to develop fully the Whole Healing System and design and orchestrate the healing process is in the end a personal endeavor. Practitioners can serve as important resources, but never as surrogate healers substituting for our own lack of initiative or commitment. The sense of the whole will be contained and situated, as it should be, within ourselves. The health continuum is liberating. It suggests that no one healer can or should master the entire healing process. It liberates the healer and researcher to study, practice, and fully develop a particular field of interest while maintaining a vision of the whole at all times. It further liberates each of us from the notion that we cannot understand or take charge of our healing. We no longer need to be victimized by the stigma of professional expertise, but can feel free to consult with practitioners while maintaining the responsibility and expertise for organizing the whole.

It may seem strange and something of an accident that a chance encounter on an airplane trip can be a source of healing for two individuals who have never previously met. But it really isn't quite that strange. Healing, as we are discovering, is ongoing and always available. Our homeostatic system is working even when we are asleep, practitioners and their therapies are ready and waiting, mind/body healing, as in this case, may be as readily accessible as the give-and-take of caring in a brief relationship, and the healing power of the spirit can be at hand instantly when we stand in awe of the simple wonders and beauty of life. Exceptional healing is merely the full use of our built-in Whole Healing System. What stands in our way is not our nature, but our allegiance to outdated ideas.

∽

INNER JOURNEYS: EXERCISING THE MIND, BODY, AND SPIRIT

Here and in the following chapters I've included a variety of exercises, or inner journeys designed to amplify the text and provide you with a direct experience of the ideas and concepts described here. The exercises can and should be repeated as many times as necessary to maximize your understanding of the text.

You may do the exercises with another person, taking turns reading to each other, or you can tape them and play them back to yourself. I have frequently added material that expands upon or reviews the concepts previously presented in the text. For some individuals, listening to such information can be an important supplement to reading it. In my practice, I suggest that the material be recorded and listened to with closed eyes.

Note the time for pauses suggested. If you are recording the exercise, simply remain silent for the indicated time. Also when reading the exercises, allow pauses between sentences to permit enough time to respond to the instructions.

~

INNER JOURNEY #1: IMAGING WHOLE HEALING

Although the material presented in this chapter is an important first step in understanding Whole Healing, a full understanding becomes possible only when we incorporate these ideas into the day-to-day fabric of our lives. In this exercise, we will complement the discussion in this chapter by presenting the same material in a way that uses your personal imagery.

Begin this exercise by allowing thirty minutes of quiet, uninterrupted time alone. Sitting comfortably in a chair, close your eyes, and allow your mind to become as still as possible.

We will begin by considering the homeostatic system. First, create the image of a person who is lying peacefully asleep. Place this image in front of your visual field. I would like you to imagine that the individual's clothes and skin are transparent, and that you can watch the inner workings of the body. Notice the normal and rhythmic pumping of the heart as it delivers the blood from the lungs to the tissues and cells of the body. Notice the thyroid, adrenal and salivary glands, automatically measuring and controlling the levels of hormones secreted in the body. Try to see the back-and-forth conversations as the body's cells communicate their needs. Notice the master gland in the brain, the pituitary gland, overseeing all of this activity. Become aware through your images of the fine balancing of minerals, blood flow, and body temperature. Notice how these activities proceed automatically and continuously while the individual is asleep. Similarly, become aware of how this system depends on the quality of the nutrients, oxygen, water, and food that the person takes in from the environment. For the next ten minutes observe how this "instinctual" automatic system self-regulates the body. At the conclusion of this period, sense how this system is working at this moment in *your* body. Why does it work in this way? What are its assets, its liabilities?

Next, let's consider the treatment system. Create an image of a practitioner's office, and an individual in the examining room. Observe how the practitioner is asking questions and examining the body for information about its workings. Observe the decision to use one or more forms of therapy: medicines, surgery, or physical therapy. For the purposes of this image let's consider that one of the forms of therapy is an antibiotic that is being used to eradicate a "strep" throat. Observe the individual purchasing the antibiotic at the pharmacy and upon arrival at home beginning ten days of medication. Watch the pill as it moves through the gastrointestinal tract, into the blood circulation, and into the tissues of the throat, where it engulfs and inactivates the bacteria. Watch how the homeostatic system assists this process by sending white blood cells to "attack" the bacteria, macrophages to "clean up" the debris, and further helps in regenerating normal tissue. Become aware, in this instance, how the homeostatic and treatment systems work together. What is the role of each? What would happen if one or the other were inactive? Allow ten minutes to complete this section of the exercise.

We will now shift to the mind/body system. Create an image of a middle-aged.man who has just suffered a heart attack and is lying in his hospital bed. By imaging the blood circulation of his heart, notice how the homeostatic system with all of its efforts cannot overcome the blockages in the coronary arteries. Some heart tissue has died, and the physicians are now injecting a medication to dissolve some of the blood clots responsible for the acute decrease in coronary blood flow. Other medications are used to control abnormal heart rhythms and maintain a normal blood pressure. While you are observing this scene, notice this individual in his normal life situation: a sixty-hour week in a highly stressful job with high demands and insufficient time or resources; a typical high-fat, quickly eaten American-type diet; insufficient time with his family to experience the nurturing and warmth of relationship. Observe how the homeostatic and treatment systems work to heal the disorder, and how the individual's life resists this effort. You may also notice how the mind/body system comes into play when the quieting of life's activities, often the result of illness, assists in focusing the body's energy on repair and healing.

Consider another image, one of a thirty-five-year-old single parent, a woman with a full-time job, two children, and unrelenting migraine headaches. Imagine the endless day-to-day activity, the absence of time for herself, of social support, or of financial security. In this instance, as in the previous one, imagine the effort to reduce stress that is made by the homeostatic system, and of the activity of the medications, treatments designed to control vascular instability. Observe how both of these systems are working against the resistance of the circumstances of this individual's life. How in each of these instances can the individual choose to activate and use the healing capacities of the

Mind/Body Healing System? Can the homeostatic and treatment systems working alone result in healing? Can you imagine in these images how and why the mind/body system has been built into the body to provide flexibility and adaptability to the Whole Healing System? Allow ten minutes.

Finally, let's consider the Spiritual Healing System. Place an image of both of these individuals in front of you. Imagine that both have now returned to their day-to-day activities with the necessary improvements in their attitudes and lifestyles. In a sense, it would be as if they were each living in a room in which they had rearranged the furniture so that the conditions were more satisfactory. Life goes on with these changes. Now consider questions these individuals ask themselves: What is the meaning of this illness, and what does it tell me about how I have been living and how I need to reorganize my life, within the limitations of my circumstances? Is there a way to view life that will bring new meaning, freshness, and vitality? How would this change my attitudes, lifestyle, and physical condition? Allow ten minutes to consider these questions as they apply to each of these individual's lives, and finally, to *yours.*

Imagine that each of the four healing systems are not separate systems, but one system with different com ponents. Create a new image of a Whole Healing System that incorporates each of the four healing systems and observe how this system moves and shifts with the movements and changes in our lives. When you are through, open your eyes.

∽

This exercise is another step in the process of learning how to see wholes rather than parts, patterns and relationships rather than separateness. Observe in your day-to-day experiences how your Whole Healing System seeks to adapt to life in a manner that is intended to heal. Allow it to lead you, to make suggestions to you, and to inform you of its needs.

ᔇ T W O ᔇ

THE CENTRE
CANNOT HOLD

Turning and turning in the widening gyre
The falcon cannot hear the falconer;
Things fall apart, the centre cannot hold;
Mere anarchy is loosed upon the world. . . .
Surely some revelation is at hand.
                              —W. B. Yeats

Recently, a conversation with a thoughtful colleague, an oncol-
ogist, illustrated to me the difficulties that arise from the assumptions of current medical practice. As we were discussing
a client I had seen that afternoon, he turned to me and said,
"The wonderful thing about science is that when you know
something has been scientifically demonstrated, you know it
can be repeated and repeated and that it will always be true." I
asked him if he thought there were other ways that truth could
be demonstrated beyond question. He quickly replied, "No." As
the conversation shifted toward his field of specialization—
cancer—he at one point quite casually stated, "You know, time
and time again I have noticed that a person who wants to live
longer, or who has a certain attitude towards cancer, or a religious faith, manages to extend his life."

"Are you sure of this?" I asked. He responded, "As sure as I am about anything."

I asked again, "Are your certain that this is true?" "Absolutely," he responded.

I pointed out to him that this was not only his observation, but an observation that has been made by many others. "But why," I asked, "can't you use this information that you know to be true the same way you use 'factual' scientifically verified information? And further, why can't we do research that further defines your understanding of the effect of attitude on the course of terminal cancer?"

"It's very difficult," he said.

He was implying that as a scientist/physician, he was neither able to place an equal value on his intuitive understandings nor comfortable using this information in his interactions with patients. For him it was beyond possibility that such knowledge could or would be considered legitimate concerns for scientific inquiry. He felt compelled to deny a personal truth, and further, to deny to both himself and his client knowledge that could potentially influence recovery and health. Rather, he chose to subordinate his truths to a biomedical model whose untested principles and assumptions he was only dimly aware of. This is the tragedy and irrationality of a model, scientific or otherwise, that denies the validity of knowledge that cannot be made to "fit" the current model.

Models can be empowering. They provide us with a clear, concise, and efficient way to interpret and respond to problems. Although we are infrequently aware of their influence, models and their underlying principles and assumptions have a powerful authority over our lives. They quietly but insistently organize the ways we perceive and respond to aspects of our lives. To the extent that models are accurate and complete, they provide effective answers to problems. When they are limited or antiquated, their effectiveness rapidly declines.

A model is an explanatory map. As a road map shows us how to travel from one place to another, an explanatory map, such as the Whole Healing model, assists us in systematically arranging our thoughts, ideas, and actions into a cohesive and consistent framework that provides direction and allows us to make sense of our inner and outer lives. If we follow an inaccurate or incomplete road map, we are unlikely to arrive at our destination. Similarly, if we follow an inaccurate or incomplete healing map, it is unlikely that we will achieve full healing. Each of the four healing systems discussed in the preceding chapter are maps that explain healing. Each one addresses a singular aspect of healing, so that taken alone each is also limited. This is why Whole Healing requires a comprehensive and integrated approach.

THE PRINCIPLES OF THE BIOMEDICAL MODEL

As a physician in training the only healing model I learned was the biomedical treatment model. At the time I was unaware, as I imagine was also the case with my instructors, of the principles (or should I say assumptions) upon which this model and my entire professional work were based. I say assumptions because I mean just that. Models are not grounded so much on fact as they are on assumptions. It is only later, when the model has been accepted, that research, based upon the model, seeks to affirm its fundamental assumptions. The biomedical model is rooted in a series of principles and assumptions, a paradigm or worldview, that slowly but assuredly emerged from the observational methods and philosophical thoughts of Copernicus, Galileo, Descartes, and Newton in the sixteenth and seventeenth centuries. The three basic, essentially *untested*, assumptions of that model are *objectivism, determinism,* and *positivism.* These three ideas have had enormous effect on how we live our lives, and particularly on how we approach issues of health and healing.

It came as a shock to me to discover that I knew very little about the origins of biomedical science, a science I had studied for many years. I had always assumed, without knowing, that its basic tenets were proven, or at best indisputable truths. I was wrong. These truths were really empirical assumptions expressing a particular historical perspective. They represented the best assumptions about the operations of nature that could be made with the knowledge available some 500 years ago. However, the assumptions emerged from the Middle Ages, a period dominated by a religious worldview. The need for a strong, empirical, sensory-based science was basic and timely. The shift resulted in the development of an extraordinary scientific understanding of life. As I began to study the origins of biomedicine, I developed a great respect for the brilliance of this model and its accomplishments, but I also became aware of its limitations and its chilling influence on all other ways of thinking and knowing.

It is impossible to overstate this last fact. Born into the world of Western science, all we have ever known is this particular way of seeing the world. We believe in it because it is familiar, culturally acceptable, and appears to explain a great deal about how things work. We trust it, and have bought into it. Tradition has a strong pull that retains what works but it also inhibits new initiatives and directions. It keeps us from questioning the status quo or whether things could be better. In Albert Einstein's words, "Concepts which have been proved to be useful in ordering things easily acquire such an authority over us that we forget their human origin and accept them as invariable."

Stop for a moment and look at the figure on the next page. What do you see? It's likely that you see two overlapping triangles. But that's not what's really there. The mind has filled in the missing lines to create a mental image that is entirely different from the actual image. Yet no matter how many times you look at it, your mental activity will attempt to fit this image into your existing thought patterns. When I asked the graphic designer to redo this graphic from a shaded gray to a white background she immediately said, "If I do that you'll lose the triangles." "That's not possible," I replied, "because the triangles are not on the paper; they're in your head." She took another look, and then laughed.

RESHAPING REALITY

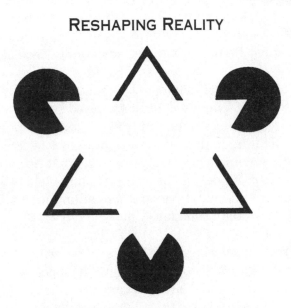

In spite of a concentrated effort, the mind will continue to see two overlapping triangles in this image. Of course they are not there. If required, our minds will reshape and distort reality, to fit it into a form that resembles our past experiences.

The mind operates by trying to make new realities fit old ways of seeing, even if this requires that it reshape and distort reality in order to conform to what we know. That's why, if we wish our new ideas to remain untainted by "what was," we must remain continuously aware of our old ways of thinking. This means that the consideration of a new view may require that we first place aside, or deconstruct, our existing viewpoint and move into the unknown. But this is neither easy nor comfortable. Consider René Magritte's painting called *Time Transfixed*.

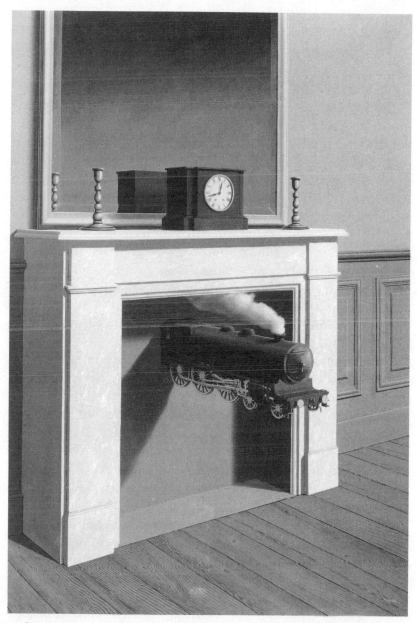

In this painting, *Time Transfixed*, the surrealist artist René Magritte presents us with an image that is meant to undermine our capacity to make sense of it through our past experiences. He is thrusting us into the unknown, and in the process is confronting us with its discomfort, confusion, and disorientation.

While looking at this image, notice the difficulty it creates for your mind. Become aware of the inner discord, confusion, and the increased mental activity as your mind, with great difficulty, flips through its memory searching for a previous experience that can help it explain this image. When it cannot, the mind uselessly persists in trying to make sense out of it. But it can't, and it's far more comfortable and easier to let this aberration go and return to the known than it is to stay with it. This is precisely why it is so difficult to change worldviews. When we experience an idea, an image, or an event that we can reshape to fit our existing perspective, such as in the example of the triangles depicted above, our minds gratefully accept whatever distortions and illusions are required. But when we cannot accomplish even that much, we find ourselves in the unknown, at sea without a compass, a choice few of us would make whatever possibilities it may open.

New ways of thinking and being shift the ground under our feet; they lead to uncertainty and discomfort. The choice we face is this: Should we transform the old, with all its comfort and reliability, into a new, revitalized, but unsure world, or should we remain as we are, limited but certain? When we do choose, fundamental change is no less than a deconstruction of one world and the construction of another. Most assuredly this can take place in small steps, yet each small step, much like the larger ones, feels risky and uncertain.

Given what we know about how the mind operates, when it comes to healing, if we want change, we need to examine the assumptions and principles that guide our choices carefully. The historic ideas of *objectivism*, *determinism*, and *positivism* represent a worldview that defines an entire way of living and being, as do the contrasting ideas of *dynamism*, *holism*, and *purposefulness*, which represent a very different perspective. The character and dimensions of our health and the very nature of our lives are largely predetermined by the choices we make among these ideas. If we are to take charge of our healing, we must first change the worldview that silently, yet very powerfully, guides our lives. As you read the descriptions of the assumptions and principles that follow, close your eyes and imagine how they operate in your life. You may be surprised.

THE PRINCIPLES AND ASSUMPTIONS OF MODERN SCIENCE

OBJECTIVISM

Objectivism is the conviction that life and nature can be best understood through the measurement of information acquired through the use of our senses. In this view, life is reduced to what we see, hear, touch, smell, and taste. This idea assumes that our thoughts and feelings have no influence on the hard realities that we observe through our senses. According to this assumption, the content of the mind is completely divorced from the recordings of the sensory system, and accurate knowledge can only be gained through "untainted," objectified sensory experience. What you see is what is there, and nothing more.

Objectivism defines two separate worlds: the world of inner experience and the "real" world of outer, sensory-based experience. Sensory-based observation and experimentation have made important contributions to our lives. Nevertheless, this perspective, when taken as an exclusive approach to knowledge, is one of the great unspoken flaws of science in general, and the biomedical model in particular. Even such an objectified field as theoretical physics has demonstrated that the observer cannot be separated from his or her observations. The choice of what we observe, the method of observation, and the framework within which we interpret our findings are already a blend of subjective experience and sensory intake. There is no singular "objective" reality. What *I* think, what *I* feel, how *I* observe, and how *I* measure are an inseparable part of what *I* experience. In physics this is called the Heisenberg principle. In medicine it is simply common sense.

But life is not the same as chemistry. It cannot be comprehended only through the accumulation of laboratory results, bacterial cultures, or X-ray examinations. Yet these printouts of an exclusively "objectified" science are the essential elements of medical diagnosis. As practitioners and individuals we learn to devalue subjective information and disregard personal experience. Data takes on a life of its own, automatically dictating our choices and actions. As practitioners we find ourselves treating lab results rather than people, and as individuals we slowly but surely assimilate this mechanistic view of ourselves.

Common sense teaches us that how we see things makes a difference, and that our thoughts, feelings, and perceptions are valid and significant sources of information even though they are neither measurable nor quantifiable in the standard ways of medical science. The idea of objectivism, which has assisted in the development of an important and reliable method of expanding knowledge, is valuable. However, when the concept of objectivism is held as an inviolable principle, it is deeply flawed because it denies the significance of the many subjective forces that shape personal experience—the complex, interwoven tapestry of our lives. The result is partial knowledge.

DETERMINISM

Determinism is the belief that an unbroken chain of events directly and inflexibly connects a specific cause to its specific effect. For example, this law would predict that (A) a genetic defect that alters the metabolism of cholesterol by necessity leads to (B) an elevation of serum cholesterol, which contributes to (C) the development of cholesterol plaques in the coronary blood vessels, which, when critically obstructed, results in (D) a blockage of blood flow, and (E) the death of the related cardiac muscle, or a heart attack.

$$A \rightarrow B \rightarrow C \rightarrow D \rightarrow E$$

According to this view, there is a direct and linear upward chain of events that is *determined* by the initial genetic abnormality (A). The implication is clear. The deterministic rule of linear upward causation requires that: (1) the cause of disease, by necessity, must occur at the biochemical level; (2) once discovered, this biochemical abnormality can be repaired; and (3) correction of this abnormality (A) will automatically reverse the upward chain of events B through E.

But let's look further at the validity of this as it applies to heart disease. Why are there individuals with high levels of serum cholesterol who exhibit no evidence of heart disease? Why can heart disease be influenced through attitudinal and lifestyle changes without altering a biochemical defect? Could it be that the cause of heart disease cannot be isolated to a single biochemical abnormality and its upward effects? We are now recognizing that this disease, as with other diseases, is a complex disorder caused in part by the upward effects of a biochemical abnormality, but also by the *downward* effects of personal attitudes and lifestyles, particularly eating habits, stress, and social isolation. The causes of heart disease are not exclusively *determined* by a linear chain of events related to one specific abnormality, but rather are the result of a unique *web* of interactive experiences that are specific to a single individual at all times.

As we have seen, the assumptions of science are pervasive. Consider the issue of causation in our own lives. We always try to find the single cause of our problems or the one issue or change that will improve life. "If only he would change," "If only

I had more money, or had chosen differently," are our constant reprises. It is far more difficult to entertain the possibility that our experiences are the result of multiple factors: our beliefs and actions, those of others, our natural temperament, nature's way of teaching us, and our body's attempts at adaptation and change. To see how patterns and interwoven events give rise to the present is neither as convenient nor as efficient as the belief in a single causative factor, but such a way of seeing may provide us with respect for the complexity of life's events, and ultimately with a more effective way of guiding our lives. The problem is that we are not accustomed to seeing in this way. We are always pulled back to single-cause thinking, a principle of science that has become a principle of life.

Determinism is one way things work, and as one approach to understanding life's events it has provided us with much valid and useful knowledge. But for humans, multiple forces, predictable and unpredictable, define the character and quality of the living experience. Among these are consciousness, volition, will, and lifestyle choices, characteristics that vary from individual to individual and that interact with biochemical factors at all times to shape the living experience cooperatively. A principle that may apply to planetary movements cannot be similarly and exclusively applied to the human condition.

POSITIVISM

Positivism is the belief that an understanding of life can only be derived from what we can see through our senses and prove through the positive and repeatable findings of scientific experiments. Stated another way, biomedical science adheres to the assumption that legitimate and accurate knowledge is exclusively and progressively constructed through the accretion of measurable and quantifiable facts. If we conduct enough experiments we will rule out those possibilities that are not verifiable facts, and slowly build a version of the truth that is based on positive experimental findings, a truth that will ultimately be life enhancing.

This approach provides us with a very specific and narrow view of truth. Yet most of us would agree that those things we know to be most true are directly learned through intuitive "aha" experiences. The idea of positivism leaves no room for knowledge that is gained through consciousness, intuitiveness, empathy, or in any way other than sensory-based experiences. How one-dimensional our world would be if it were exclusively composed of what can be discovered through our senses. Can trust, love, compassion, or hope be measured, quantified, seen, touched, or otherwise positively demonstrated? If not, does this mean that they neither exist nor have significant impact on our minds and bodies? The scientific assumption of positivism, often unknown to practitioners or clients, severely limits the information that can be legitimately considered when a symptom or disorder is assessed and a therapeutic plan is proposed. The results of experimental science, the acquisition of sensory-based information, provides us with an important way of understanding life. Nevertheless, it is only one way of understanding human experience.

THE PRINCIPLES OF BIOMEDICINE

Objectivism	The conviction that life and nature can be most accurately understood through sensory based information.
Determinism	The conviction that an unbroken chain of events directly and inflexibly links a prior singular cause to its specific effect.
Positivism	The conviction that an understanding of life and nature are exclusively derived from sensory-based observations and the positive and repeatable findings of scientific experimentation.

The principles that are responsible for the development of biomedical science are significant and valid, but they are *partial truths*. Biomedical science, as a *singular* approach to healing, is quite limited. Its increasingly apparent limitations are now driving the development of a more comprehensive approach to healing, an approach that calls for a new and broader set of assumptions.

THE PRINCIPLES AND ASSUMPTIONS OF WHOLE HEALING

The principles of Whole Healing, *dynamism, holism,* and *purposefulness*, are not different from the assumptions underlying the biomedical model in that they are ideas created with the human mind for the purpose of understanding and effectively dealing with life. The difference lies in the fact that these principles allow us greater freedom, flexibility, and possibility than the biomedical principles because they are based on a more comprehensive vision of healing, one that is appropriate to our time, our consciousness, and our needs. Let's examine each of these principles.

DYNAMISM

Dynamism, or change, growth, and development, is the quality of a living organism that is at all times in an active and vital relationship with its environment, continuously exchanging information and nutrients and adaping to new and different circumstances. As living organisms, humans are open systems. In contrast, biomedical science views man as a closed system. Closed systems, like machines, are highly predictable because once they are set in motion they cannot change. For example, if a series of chemicals is added to a flask and the flask is closed, the end stage of the solution, the result of the chemical interactions, is known from the initial conditions. What we initially place in the flask exclusively determines the outcome. Machines are similar. Once they are put together they work in a predictable and unchanging way. We now know that this is a very limited understanding of the human condition.

Human life is characterized by both a built-in set of physiological activities that assure survival and the capacity to adapt, within limits, to new conditions. Adaptation is influenced by consciousness and its choice of perspectives, attitudes, lifestyles, and environments. As a result, as humans we are open systems capable of continuously changing, destroying, and re-creating ourselves. In a sense, our bodies regularly dissolve and regenerate, and under ideal conditions our consciousness would do much the same as it attends to each present moment. This ongoing creative process is what distinguishes animate from inanimate life. In contrast, the principles of biomedicine are static; they do not address the property of dynamism and change. At its core, human life is an ever-evolving, interactive, developmental process.

As we have discussed, the destiny of a closed system is determined by the initial circumstances of that system. A machine works the way it was built, will always do so, and will never change on its own. In an open system, the end point may be the same, but there are many different paths to that end point. Although all human life ends in death, we will each live our lives in very different ways. Our final fate may be equal, but the process of life provides many choices and options, or said in another way, side roads, highways, detours, and alternate routes. Healing becomes more than a single formula dictated by the accumulation of "data" and algorithmiclike therapeutic programs. It is a flexible set of options that are based on the specific and unique circumstances of any one moment in time.

HOLISM

Holism is the term we use to express the viewpoint that human life is a natural, organized, unfolding process that consists of constituent elements bound together from the very beginning as a unitary, interactive whole. As living beings we evolved from an organizational blueprint that was completely intact and operational at the time of conception. This blueprint precedes and organizes the process of differentiation and specialization, which gives rise to the molecules, cells, tissues, and organ systems in each of us. Further, it is likely that each cell in the body retains the memory and patterning of the whole (the holographic principle). A machine can neither organize itself nor, once organized, continue to develop, regenerate, and repair itself. Humans can.

Consider what it would be like to homogenize an embryo into its constituent parts. You would have a "soup" containing all of its intact components—DNA, RNA, and all the rest. If life were a machine, we could reassemble the parts into an identically functioning embryo. However, would anyone suggest that we could reconstitute a living embryo from this embryonic "soup"? From the perspective of an analytic science that postulates that life evolved over millions of years as a result of the random and blind interactions of chemical elements, the answer would be yes. If life is indeed assembled in this piecemeal manner, then with enough study and effort we should be able to learn how to reassemble the individual parts into a living whole. Theoretically, all we would need is the DNA, the correct enzymes, hormones, and sufficient know-how to create a human life. This sounds more like the script for a horror movie than an accurate description of the living process.

Let me stop here and relate to you another conversation with my physician colleague, who, it is important to point out, also has a Ph.D. in biochemistry. Attempting to explore the issue of wholes and parts somewhat further, I presented him with the experiment described above, the issue of whether the homogenized components of an embryo could be reconstituted into a living embryo. "Of course not," he said. "The genetic material, DNA, must be part of an intact cell if it is to direct the organization of the living entity." "Then," I said, "the existence of DNA is not enough; something more must be required." He agreed with this point but could not define what further factor was necessary because none of the individual cellular components by themselves or combinations of them could create an organized living form.

He did admit that this factor was clearly a quality of the living cell, and that the knowledge of the whole must be present from the beginning, preceding and directing the development of the parts. We further agreed that this factor, which has at different times been called "the vital force," "entelechy," and "the divine seed," remains more of a mystery and metaphysical issue than an appropriate subject of scientific study. "It would seem to me," I ventured, "that given what we have said, the whole must be as important to understand and work with as the parts." He replied, "I know that's true, but when I'm with patients I always seem to end up focusing on the parts, the cells and tissues that seem abnormal." I expressed sympathy with a problem I know only too well. No one could argue with our indoctrination in the assumptions of the biomedical model. We ended our conversation by agreeing that an exclusive preoccupation with the parts provided us with only a partial understanding of life and a limited capacity for healing.

I am acutely aware of how these two ways of exploring life play themselves out in my professional life. There are days when I enter the consultation room unfocused and deenergized. At such times I can feel how automatically I shift to focusing exclusively on parts, a technique that, when it becomes a well-practiced habit, requires minimal attention or energy. Work of this sort is usually brief, "disease-centered," limited, and deficient. The individual is seen mechanistically and my resources are best considered as "tools." This is in sharp contrast to those times when I approach individuals with a respect for the complexity and wholeness of human life. At such times I am able to flow back and forth between parts and wholes as I construct with the individual an understanding of the specific problem within the context of its meaning and its implications for a "larger" life. The outcome is a conscious and energizing process of Whole Healing.

PURPOSEFULNESS

Purposefulness, intentionality, and goal-directed activity can be found at every level of the human experience. A machine is not directed toward any specific goal or purpose. It performs a predesignated task, a fixed function, without reflection, development, or the capacity to reorganize itself. This is neither the fate nor the intention of human life. A fertilized egg already has within itself the pattern and blueprint that purposefully directs the entire process of human development. Purposefulness is a pervasive characteristic of human life: The automatic mechanisms of the Homeostatic Healing System aim at the maintenance of a steady state. The organ systems, the brain, and the immune, hormonal, and cardiovascular systems exhibit a capacity for memory, intelligence, and a built-in adaptability that similarly suggest purpose and direction.

What is the intention and goal of human life that seems built into our nature? This central question has occupied the minds and work of philosophers and religious leaders for centuries. As humans we are clearly a continuum rooted in the material and extending outward toward the immaterial, what some would call the divine. We are bound to automatic inner mechanisms that sustain survival, and are simultaneously provided with a capacity for awareness and consciousness that allow us to be cocreators in the evolutionary process. Thus we are built to experience the full range of possibilities that extend from tangible to intangible, from the survival of our bodies to the transcendent understanding of the sources and essence of our beings.

It makes a difference whether I view a man as a machine-like time-limited experiment of nature or whether I view him as an organized, purposeful, and meaningful expression of nature who can love, create, and have faith in his world and in his capacity to grow, change, and direct his life. The image I hold defines the character of my own life and the boundaries of my capacity as a healer. In the first view, I am limited to maintenance and structural repair, the work of a scientist/technician. In the second view, I can include these repairs in a larger vision of healing that respects the full intention of human life as it unfolds in any one person. This second view is the work of a physician/humanist. In the first instance I am involved in a brief problem-oriented encounter; in the second instance I am empathically involved in the creation of an individual's life journey.

THE PRINCIPLES OF WHOLE HEALING

Dynamism
The conviction that human life is characterized by continuous growth, development, and change.

Holism
The conviction that human life is a natural, organized, unfolding process that consists of constituent elements bound together from the very beginning as a unitary, interactive whole.

Purposefulness
The conviction that intentionality and goal-directed activity can be found at every level of the human experience.

These three principles, *dynamism*, *holism*, and *purposefulness*, form the basis for a new vision of Whole Healing. Although the principles of biomedicine and other treatment systems may continue to serve a particular aspect of healing, they must remain subservient to and integrated into a broader approach whose principles serve to encourage a more comprehensive approach to life and nature. These principles will redefine the education of practitioners, the nature of medical practice, conventional and alternative, the roles of professionals and laypeople, the domain and direction of health-insurance initiatives, and the substance and character of medical research.

Changing paradigms is not easy. In his book *The Structure of Scientific Revolutions*, Thomas Kuhn suggests that paradigms begin to change as the younger members of society and a profession, those who are less invested in the existing approaches, begin to think in new ways. The full shift may not occur until the adherents of the existing paradigm either die or become inactive in their professional lives. As a practitioner in midlife, I myself am keenly aware of how difficult and profound it is to shift one's thinking process. It is one thing to say I am a "holistic" healer; it is another to be one in the fullest sense of what it means.

Because it is rare for a complete shift in worldviews to occur within a single generation, it is helpful to return to history to catch a glimpse of what such a shift actually looks like. Consider the following images: first, the Greek sculpture called *Kouros*, 615–590 B.C., and then the *Attic Funeral Stele*, circa 330–320 B.C. In the first sculpture man is depicted as solid, mechanical, devoid of feelings, emotions, and personality. In the second sculpture, there is a vitality and humanity in the representation that is almost palpable. You can see for yourself the extraordinary shift in the way man viewed himself, a shift that occurred over the brief period of 200 years.

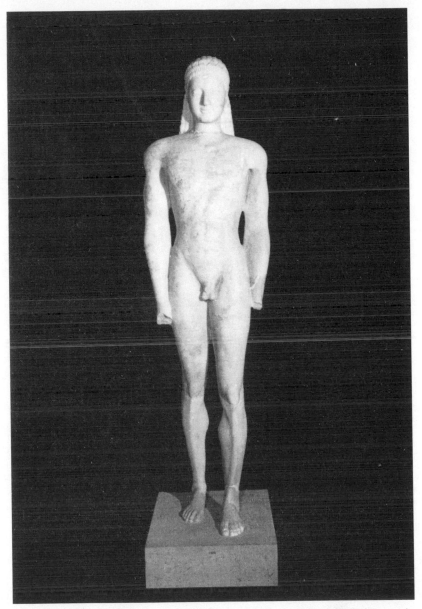

This ancient Greek kouros depicts man's view of himself in the early sixth century B.C. The figure appears mechanical, lifeless, and devoid of personality or emotions.

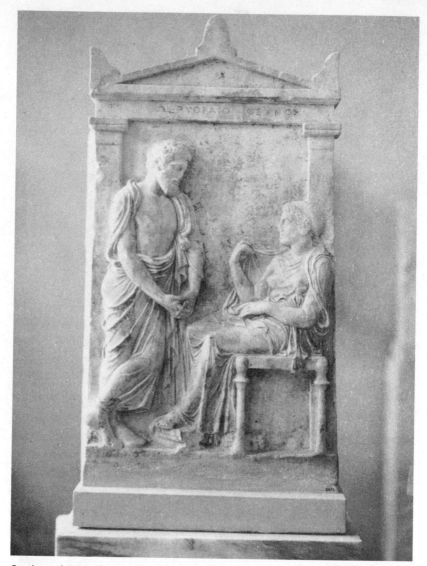

Sculpted 300 years after the kouros, this figure portrays an entirely different view of man, one that is vital and filled with individuality, emotion, and thoughtfulness. These two images of Greek sculpture reflect a profound shift in worldview.

We are each part of the next great shift in worldviews. And as a result, we live in "in-between" times, times of great discord and times of unimagined possibilities. This is now how it is with healing—one great tradition and worldview is giving way to another. The old centre cannot hold, and a revelation is surely at hand.

❦

INNER JOURNEY #2:
THE TWO STREAMS OF KNOWLEDGE

As we discussed in this chapter, we can acquire knowledge about ourselves and our world in two fundamental ways: sensory-based knowledge and nonsensory, intuitive knowledge. It is rare that a society equally accepts both. In our time, sensory-based knowledge, particularly gained through science, is the more highly valued explanation of life. But one form of knowledge unbalanced by the other is incomplete and partial. This exercise is designed to assist you in gaining a better understanding of these two ways of knowing.

Sitting comfortably in a chair, close your eyes. Imagine that there is something wrong in your life, a strange sense of discord, perhaps some fatigue or an unusual feeling that encourages you to visit your physician for an examination and evaluation. After the routine measurements of your temperature, blood pressure, and weight, you meet with your physician in his or her office. He or she asks a series of questions about the different body systems, about the appearance of unusual pain, lumps, or other unexpected physical disturbances. Your physician next leads you into the examination room and proceeds with the examination: listening to your heart and lungs, feeling your abdomen, looking in your ears and mouth, checking your reflexes, and perhaps recording an electrocardiogram, performing a breast, rectal, or gynecological examination. At the conclusion of the examination blood and urine tests are taken.

When you return for your follow-up visit, the physician informs you that according to the examination and your laboratory tests you are healthy. However, you tell your doctor you don't feel healthy. At this critical moment you and your physician, knowingly or not, are facing the limitations of sensory-based knowledge. Consider this as you remain seated with the doctor in the office. Using his or her sensory system, the physician has seen, heard, touched, and examined all that is possible. Your doctor has extended his or her direct senses to include the results of blood and urine testing. According to the accumulated data, everything is normal; of this there can be no doubt. Your physician is telling the truth. To go further with your concerns, he or she would have to step out of this form of thinking and shift to a non-sensory-based exploration of your distress. This would be to shift away from science as we know it, and more specifically for the physician, to step out of his or her training into the unknown.

For a moment, let's imagine that the physician in front of you is being transformed into a healer who has access to all forms of knowledge. He or she uses sensory-based information, but is equally comfortable with nonsensory-based knowledge, which for him or her is equally real. This new healer feels free to ask you questions about meaning, purpose, and faith, questions you about your satisfaction at work and the quality of your relationships. He or she asks you to close your eyes, and to imagine the distress you are feeling. The healer asks you to make a visual image of this distress, to place it in front of your visual field, and then examine it and ask questions of it. As you do this, you are having a more personal relationship with your distress, and more, you are trusting knowledge that is acquired from within, knowledge that cannot be quantified or measured. At the conclusion of this exploration you briefly discuss what you have learned, and your physician asks you to continue this process, returning in a week with further information that you have gathered from this inner exploration.

When you return a week later, your physician summarizes with you both the sensory-based findings of the physical examination and the information you have gained from your inner exploration. Together you arrive at a comprehensive understanding of both the physical condition of your body and its relationship to the patterns and directions of your inner life. This is not a physical examination or health appraisal in the usual sensory based way, but an assessment of all the issues in your life, mind, body, and spirit.

Without judgment, I would like you to see clearly how each of these two different legitimate sources of knowledge provides an understanding of different aspects of your life. Separately they are both limited; together they provide a comprehensive understanding, one that can lead to a plan for Whole Healing. When you are done reflecting on this, open your eyes and reorient yourself to your surroundings.

∽

Because of our cultural perspectives, it is quite difficult to accord to nonsensory-based knowledge the same significance and legitimacy accorded to sensory-based knowledge. This is for no reason other than our societal norms. One kind of knowledge is no less valuable or true than the other. These sources of knowledge are like a sheet of paper, with two sides. You cannot have an accurate and comprehensive understanding of life and nature without these two sources of knowledge. This is why we must fundamentally change our exclusive reliance on the principles and assumptions of science in a way that incorporates nonsensory-based knowledge. This is the foundation of Whole Healing.

THE HOMEOSTATIC HEALING SYSTEM

Where is the Life we have lost in living?
Where is the wisdom we have lost in knowledge?
Where is the knowledge we have lost in information?
—T. S. Eliot

The homeostatic system operates through the automatic activation of an array of internal checks and balances that assure that the body functions in a manner that can sustain life. It is our gift at birth. It is nature at its most elegant, yet also at its most simple. It can take a lifetime to appreciate its wisdom and to learn to get out of its way. It is our most direct connection to the primal forces of nature. When the homeostatic system detects a deviation from "normal," it automatically rebalances our physiology by activating a balancing mechanism, which returns the body to its routine operating conditions.

Homeostasis works through built-in feedback loops, which are guided by an innate intelligence and knowledge that have been gained from the millennia of human experience, a sort of extended process of learning through trial and error. For example, the homeostatic system maintains salt and water balance, regulates blood pressure and pulse within narrow limits, and stabilizes our clotting mechanisms in a manner that sustains the fluidity of our blood, yet, when necessary, it automatically activates our coagulation mechanisms to patch any leaks.

To carry out its routine activities the homeostatic system requires the conditions, physiological and psychological, that will support its operations. It is a conservative system that slowly adapts to changing human conditions. As noted in Chapter 1, it may take 1 million years to achieve a 5 percent change in the way our bodies work. Compare our fast-paced urban life, a recent event in human history, to the primitive conditions under which our biology developed. As we are now discovering, our modern and urban lifestyles, attitudes, and physical and social environments are often alien to and disruptive of our homeostatic mechanisms. These four factors may contribute up to 70 percent of the underlying sources of the top 10 fatal diseases, and they play an equally significant role in the stress and degenerative disorders that, although often nonfatal, account for considerable distress and disability.

Thus, when an individual such as Dan, a young college student with complaints of increasingly frequent and severe headaches, first visits my office I mentally run through the four healing systems and decide which to approach first. Most of the time I start by addressing the basic homeostatic needs of the mind and body: the need for a nutritious diet, exercise, sleep, healthy attitudes, and supportive relationships, each of which is essential for the optimal function of the Homeostatic Healing System. These are not "high-tech" issues, and for some individuals they may seem somewhat irrelevant, or at best of minor significance. But they are potent sources of healing that can realign our lives with the long-evolved needs of our minds and bodies. I am amazed at how few of us get regular and adequate sleep, a necessity for a well-functioning immune system, or exercise, which helps to condition the heart, regulate blood-sugar levels, and maintain normal blood pressure. I am always distressed, but unfortunately not surprised, by my patients' lack of supportive and nurturing relationships, which, as we shall discuss later, are essential to a healthy life, or the absence of time alone, an ingredient of a balanced mind. These are not luxuries; they are instinctual needs. We deny these needs at great cost. In Dan's case, the cost was a breakdown of the homeostatic system, a breakdown that resulted in his painful headaches.

The internal and automatic homeostatic system is the grand result of evolution's ongoing experiment with life. To "listen" to its wisdom is to discern the way nature means us to live. When we violate this long-developed covenant with nature, our minds and bodies inform us of this by providing the signs and symptoms of physical and emotional imbalance. Seen from this perspective, disease, particularly the epidemics of stress and degenerative disease, is a dramatic indicator of the distance we have traveled from our early communion with nature, a progressive estrangement that cannot be remedied by treatments alone.

CHECKS AND BALANCES: THE BODY'S AUTOPILOT

Fortunately for each of us, our physiology is largely automated and directed by the monitoring and balancing mechanisms of the Homeostatic Healing System, which is built in. Left to themselves, the mechanisms do quite well, but human consciousness, particularly when it is undeveloped, too often exhibits its arrogance by arranging circumstances and living conditions for which these mechanisms are ill suited. The result can usually be seen in a practitioner's office, where treatment is sought. Treatment systems (of which biomedicine is the foremost in our culture) are developed to remedy the inability of the homeostatic system to adapt successfully to the stressful and unhealthy conditions of modern life. In our eagerness to outdo nature, we often forget to consider our natural self-healing mechanisms.

Recently, an article appearing in *The New England Journal of Medicine* reemphasized the need to support the Homeostatic Healing System. For decades it has been medical practice to rapidly replace fluid loss in individuals whose blood pressure has precipitously dropped as a result of severe blood loss due to trauma. The rationale for this approach is based on the view that rapid rehydration elevates the blood pressure toward normal, allowing for better perfusion to the body's essential organs prior to surgery. It makes sense, doesn't it?

Perhaps to our logical minds, but not to the body. Consider the possibility that the automatic lowering of blood pressure following the rapid loss of blood may be a normal compensatory mechanism of the body, a normal homeostatic response that has meaning and purpose. If this were so, we would listen more carefully and trust the wisdom of the body, and then reconsider our approach in these cases. The results of such an experiment were reported in the *Journal* article.

In this large hospital study individuals entering the emergency room with acute trauma and reduced blood pressure from blood loss were divided into two groups. One group received fluid administration prior to surgery and the other did not. To everyone's surprise, the group that did not receive fluid replacement had a higher survival rate, and left the hospital earlier. It seems that somewhere in human history the body had figured out how to handle rapid blood loss effectively long before we developed intravenous therapy. Maintaining a lower blood pressure under these conditions allows the blood to form clots more easily, which can further retard blood loss, and once formed, these clots are more resistant to dislodgment because of the diminished blood pressure. This is only one example of how treatment can interfere with the innate intelligence of the body by failing to use its basic healing mechanisms.

We interfere with the normal maintenance and healing capacities of the body in many other ways. For example, the high-fat diets characteristic of Western society are far from the nutritional environment in which the homeostatic system evolved. Fats are responsible for the plaques that occlude our arteries, for the vascular instability that leads to an excessive vascular tone, an effect that contributes to heart disease and to the development of certain types of cancer. Unfortunately, we have yet to document fully how our diet has confused our sophisticated physiological mechanisms, which evolved on a high-fiber low-fat diet.

For example, in the 1970s a British epidemiologist, D. Burkitt, discovered while studying the native diets of Africans that our high-fat diets, diets that substitute fat for fiber, have resulted in a uniquely Western disease called diverticulosis. It seems that diverticulosis, small outpocketings of the colon that increase with age, result from a lifelong alteration in the muscular activity of the bowel. This alteration is a consequence of the absence of high levels of fiber in our diet, a shift that began in the mid to late nineteenth century when milling techniques were developed to remove increasing amounts of fiber from flour and when alternate food sources became available. Since Burkitt's observation, dietary fiber has become a standard of treatment for this disorder, a disorder that is unknown in cultures that have retained their traditional dietary patterns. Burkitt also noted that in communities in which diverticulosis was rare, "so were benign polyps, and the incidence of cancer of the colon and of ulcerative colitis." There is also an association between diverticula and cardiovascular disease, duodenal ulcer, appendicitis, and diabetes. Here again we see how lifestyle changes that fail to establish and support the conditions for the normal functioning of the homeostatic system give rise to the diseases of modern life.

Much the same can be said about the body's need for exercise, clean water, and clean air. The development of urban life has significantly altered these vital conditions, conditions present at the time our homeostatic system developed. Poorly adapted to living under these changed circumstances, we suffer from stress-related disease and chronic degenerative disorders that are unique to modern man. It is fair to say that there are things over which we have minimal control, such as air and water quality, but the point is that there are many other ways we can support and encourage homeostatic healing merely by attending to some of the basic built-in needs of the body. A high-fiber low-fat diet, exercise, sound sleep, plentiful relationships, and healthy attitudes are the concerns that should be at the top of a homeostatic healing program.

SOUND MIND, SOUND BODY

The physiological conditions under which we prosper, conditions under which the homeostatic system can optimally function, are naturally linked to psychological conditions. To understand this linkage between the mind and body, we turn to the emerging field of scientific investigation called psychoneuroimmunology (PNI). PNI brings together three previously separate areas of inquiry: psychology, the study of behavior; neurology, the study of the brain; and immunology, the study of the body's natural defense system. PNI provides us with an understanding of the recently discovered mechanics of the mind/body connection, and although these interactions occur automatically (this is to say that the mind and body are routinely communicating with each other for the purpose of maintaining a mind/body balance), we can also activate and direct them with intention. In this way these same mechanisms can serve the Mind/Body Healing System (which we will discuss shortly).

We have known for a long time about two of the links that connect the mind and body: the autonomic nervous system, a series of nerves that link the nervous system to many of the body organs, and the central nervous system, which controls gross motor function, the movement of our arms and legs. The breakthrough to new knowledge came when Candace Pert, an early PNI researcher, uncovered a previously unknown link, a third communication system made up of a group of protein-based messenger chemicals called neuropeptides. The neuropeptide messenger system differs from the autonomic and central nervous systems in two important ways. First, the neuropeptide system is not fixed in place; it is a mobile communication system that moves freely, by way of blood circulation, throughout the body. Second, we now know that the messenger chemicals are not only synthesized by brain cells, but by many other cells in the body, and are therefore part of a twenty-four-hour bidirectional communication system that links all aspects of the brain with all aspects of the body.

Scientists have identified more than sixty different neuropeptides that serve as messenger chemicals moving information back and forth throughout the mind and body. They are seeing an ongoing conversation between cells that is mediated by the neuropeptide messenger system. These discoveries make it increasingly difficult to distinguish either mind from body or emotions from sensations. In Candace Pert's words, "The mind is the body. The body is the mind." Neuropeptides, the messenger chemicals, are produced in response to thoughts, feelings, and images; they shift the physiology of the body to correspond to the specific state of the mind. Nature, it seems, has meant to include the entire human experience, physiology and psychology, in its homeostatic plan of maintaining balance. And it appears to have done so largely through the intermediary of the neuropeptide messenger system.

What are the psychological factors that interact with our physiology to promote homeostasis, a balanced body? Aaron Antonovsky, a noted medical sociologist, has studied aspects of this specific question. The focus of his work was to explore and uncover the psychological factors that promote health and simultaneously increase our resistance to disease. He called these characteristics *salutogenic* factors, health-inducing factors or as we may call them, homeostatic balancing factors. Through interviews with selected individuals he was able to identify three constant and central psychological qualities that seem to characterize individuals in whom the homeostatic sys-

tem appears to work at an optimal level. Together these qualities convey to the individual what he called *a sense of coherence*, or a sense of balance and integrity.

According to Antonovsky, the three psychological markers
of a sense of coherence are manageability, comprehensibility,
and meaningfulness. Let's look at each of these separately.
Manageability is an individual's sense that he or she has access to the resources and capacities to meet life's problems
successfully. This consists of both a feeling of trust in the effectiveness of one's capacities and the actual availability of
skills and resources. *Comprehensibility* is the belief that
things make sense, that it is possible to understand why things
happen as they do. *Meaningfulness* is the capacity to see the
events and experiences of life (adversity included) as having
meaning, purpose, and direction.

Suzanne Kobassa, a clinical researcher in the field of PNI,
approached the question of homeostasis from a somewhat different direction. She surveyed a group of middle- and upper-
level executives at a large public utility with the aim of
identifying two distinct groups: individuals reporting high
stress and high illness, and those reporting high stress and low
illness, that is, those whose systems were out of balance and
those who managed to maintain balance under the very same
external conditions. She asked each group to complete a series of questionnaires directed at uncovering any psychological qualities or characteristics that could account for the
apparent protection from stress-related disease that was ob-
served in the second group. She called these personality qualities *hardiness*. Kobassa found that the executives with high
stress/low illness shared three personality characteristics or
attitudes that were lacking in the high stress/high illness
group: commitment, control, and a sense of challenge.

Kobassa concluded that a *commitment to self* reflected a
clear sense of one's values, goals, and capabilities, as well as a
belief in their importance. It is knowing "who I am and what
my life is about." *A sense of control*, as it implies, resulted from

the ability to maintain a feeling of control that results from responding to life's experiences in a manner that is direct, forceful, and resourceful. A *sense of challenge* describes the vigorousness with which such individuals approach life and its many experiences. For such individuals, adversity is seen as a potential opportunity, a time for new initiatives.

SENSE OF COHERENCE	HARDINESS
Manageability: access to resources and capacities to meet life's problems	Commitment to Self: clear sense of values, goals, capabilities
Comprehensibility: belief that things make sense	Sense of Control: ability to maintain a feeling of control in responding to life's circumstances
Meaningfulness: capacity to see events as having meaning and purpose	Sense of Challenge: adversity is seen as opportunity and challenge

The chart above summarizes the specific psychological qualities that Antonovsky and Kobassa have linked to our physiology, qualities that promote health and enhance our resistance to disease. Note how similar their findings are. These psychological factors create the essential psychic context for homeostasis. They can serve to buffer stress and thereby support the healthy functioning of the homeostatic system. These qualities that support our natural healing system, unlike physiological factors, are not built in. In fact, urban life more often promotes the opposite qualities: helplessness, powerlessness, and estrangement. So what we are discovering is that urban life requires us to bring into play healing systems other than homeostatis or treatment, in this case the Mind/Body Healing System, which we will discuss in detail below. In this way we develop the psychological qualities that will support and enhance the routine balancing activities of the ancient homeostatic system whose function is compromised by the inhospitable conditions of modern life.

THE IMPORTANCE OF THE OTHER

Our social life, as well as our psychological life, is part of the seamless experience of the human condition. That is, change any one aspect of life, our social life, psychology, or physiology, and every other aspect also changes. As we shall see in more detail in Chapter 7, an extensive volume of incontestable research documents the relationship of health and longevity to an individual's level of social integration, i.e., one's propensity to affiliate with others in marriage, church, community activities, work, and friendships. There is clearly something about relationships that is health sustaining, and similarly, in the case of dysfunctional relationships or loss of a loved one, detrimental to health. Healthy social relationships support homeostasis.

Consider the following. Michael G. Marmot, a medical researcher, studied the changing incidence of coronary heart disease among recent Japanese immigrants to the United States as compared with residents of Japan. He found that the incidence of heart disease was lowest in Japan, intermediate in Hawaii, and highest in California. This difference could not be explained solely on the basis of differences in the customary risk factors: dietary intake, serum cholesterol levels, blood pressure, or smoking. To analyze the findings further, Marmot carefully examined the California sample. There he discovered that Japanese men who were *most acculturated to Western society* (most separated from their traditional culture) had three to five times more heart disease than those Japanese who retained much of their traditional values and practices.

Marmot suggests that close traditional family ties and the

low incidence of Type A behavior (urgency, competitiveness, and hostility) serve to protect the Japanese from developing heart disease. As these social relationships change and long-held traditions give way to social conditions that are adverse to the coherence of the Japanese family and its customs, we see a proportionate rise in the incidence of disease (in this report, heart disease). A similar rise in the incidence of disease can be seen in other cases of social disruption: the plight of refugees, the rise of unemployment rates, disruptive marital relationships, and the loss of a spouse.

Social relationships are a very important issue in the day-to-day practice of medicine. The death of a spouse, the loss of an important relationship, disharmony in relationships, and the upheaval of moving from one town to another often precede the onset of illness—a fact I can readily testify to from my years of medical practice. People are healthier and recover more quickly from illness when they have friends, family, and other supportive relationships that are both consistent and reliable. There is something very primal about the manner in which our healthy social interactions, emotional bonding, caring, touching, and the other aspects of relationship interact with our physiology and psychology to sustain an inner balance. At a time when our relationships to each other and to our communities are strained and many of us are experiencing increasing levels of estrangement and alienation, it is essential to remind ourselves that our physiology "grew up" in stable, traditional communities with a constant support group and familiar surroundings.

NAVIGATING THE HOMEOSTATIC HEALING SYSTEM

At first glance the homeostatic system seems to require little attention. It appears to carry out its physiological functions quietly and automatically, maintaining with ease the inner milieu that is essential for life. But at second glance we see a very different story. Working under conditions far different from the original conditions required by these autoregulatory mechanisms, they can no longer guarantee either survival or effective self-healing. But to ignore the power and wisdom of this system is only to commit ourselves to further, more complicated efforts at treatment, even while built into the mind and body, waiting for us to use it, is our first and most natural capacity for healing.

Where do we begin? How do we help to activate and maximize the healing power of the Homeostatic Healing System? We begin by learning to do what comes quite naturally to this system: sensing the mind and body and becoming keenly aware of any imbalances. To be aware of our minds and bodies, to know what is happening and what is needed, can be as simple as recognizing and acknowledging fatigue before exhaustion sets in, stress before it results in body breakdown, and early discomfort before it reflects itself in the signs and symptoms of disease. Then we can react with the appropriate response, which might be staying home from work and crawling into bed when feeling ill rather than seeking martyrdom at the office, adding further rest and time alone when we are fatigued or overstressed, and attending to the subtle changes that indicate a growing imbalance and disharmony. Because we are conscious beings we have the capacity either to get in the way of our natural homeostatic tendencies or to encourage and support them.

It always amazes me that individuals expect me to know more about their minds and bodies than they do themselves. For example, I cannot count the number of times I have asked individuals who are complaining of headaches the following question: "What occurred within the three- to six-month period preceding the onset of the headaches that could have been related to them?" The answer is usually "Nothing that I can think of." Here is an individual, suffering for months, who is unable to make this cause-and-effect association. I know that if I persist with my questioning, I will almost always discover what in retrospect is an obvious psychological or social life event that has occurred contemporaneously with the onset of the symptom and is clearly the source of the problem.

Only recently I received a telephone call from the mother of a college student asking that I arrange for an MRI of her daughter's brain during Christmas break, an evaluation that had been recommended by her daughter's college physician, who had been considering her recent headaches. I requested that the daughter visit me first. When I asked Susan whether she could relate any event to these headaches, she proclaimed, "No, nothing has happened to cause these, they just began without any reason." Although it was the end of a tiring day, I began to probe. She didn't make it easy, but at one point, with extreme casualness, she mentioned that she had recently ended a long-term relationship with a high school sweetheart. "No big deal," she said. "I'm finished with it." She then went on to the next thought. It was then that I knew the source of her headaches. The fact that I knew it before she knew it was significant. One doesn't end a long intimate relationship, particularly one's first love, without grief. As we began to speak about this she revealed that she habitually suppresses her feelings. What an understatement! Not only did she hide her emotions from others, she hid them from herself. Feelings, when unacknowledged, express themselves through the body. She is now back in college, absent a $1,000 MRI, attending counseling sessions and learning about the expression of grief and other emotions.

Grieving and the expression of feelings are normal homeostatic healing mechanisms. If we allow the mechanisms to function as they were designed to function, the healing will be automatic; when we block it, we court breakdown and distress. All we did about Susan's headaches was to assess the problem and set in motion a process that would allow for homeostatic healing. *We did not heal through our discovery of the source of the headaches or through the counseling, but rather, we established the conditions for the mind and body to self-heal; we activated and facilitated the Homeostatic Healing System.* And often this is all we have to do. The mind and body know how to heal. If we can figure out how we have gotten in the way, we can reestablish the conditions for natural healing.

Consider another example. Mike arrived in my office complaining of fatigue, stomach distress, and sleeplessness. He had already decided that the solution was a potent antacid tablet and a sleeping pill, two of the fastest-selling drugs on the market. As we talked further, he told me about his recent move from another state, his frantic weekend efforts to travel back and forth to visit his girlfriend, and the unexpected stress of his new job. His system had been completely thrown off by the move: the disruption of his relationship, the pressures of a new job, and the loss of his support network that had remained in his hometown. Any reasonable person, including Mike, could see that none of these problems require a pill, or for that matter diagnostic testing. Our conversation and the beginning of our relationship itself served to heal the sources of his distress. Once we identified the problem, the solutions were easy to find. Mike's girlfriend began to do more of the traveling, he joined a hiking group, we met more frequently, and he had an extended talk with his new supervisor. We identified the sources of his imbalance and initiated very simple actions that would support the homeostatic needs of his mind and body.

Whether we are dealing with a headache, an ulcer, stress, fatigue, or any other symptom, if we have lost the ability to sense the impending dysfunction early in its course, we have simultaneously lost the capacity to support our homeostatic healing systems. To support the homeostatic system effectively we must develop the capability of sensing imbalance, recognizing its sources, and initiating effective compensatory actions, physical, psychological, or social. We can wait for the overt signs and symptoms of distress or, far better, proactively support the needs of our homeostatic systems.

As we have seen, the basics are exercise, healthy nutrition, appropriate sleep, a clean environment, the psychological qualities of *hardiness* and *coherence*, and healthy social relationships. Beyond this, a careful and close attention to our minds and bodies will inform us of our specific needs at any one moment. We have noted that a system that earlier in time was automatic, now, given our estrangement from the living conditions of our ancestors, requires our active support and cooperation. We no longer can view homeostasis as merely a static, self-directing automatic healing system. We must now begin to understand how we can actively engage and enhance this extraordinary natural healing system.

ᕲᕮ

INNER JOURNEY #3: SENSING MIND/BODY BALANCE

Becoming aware of the subtle rhythms and movements of the mind and body is what will allow us to shift our attitudes, lifestyles, and environments in a direction that will support the self-healing potential of the homeostatic system. The intuitive questions we should learn to ask are, Am I in balance or out of balance? Do my mind and body have what they need, or not? We are masters at outer sensitivity, reacting almost instantaneously to approval or rejection, success or failure. We must similarly become masters at inner sensitivity, reacting as quickly to readjust our circumstances when we feel an imbalance or a disturbance of the natural feeling of peace and health.

Find a comfortable spot and either sit or lie down with your eyes closed. Allow a few moments for the thoughts, feelings, and images of the past few minutes to move out of awareness. You may take several full deep breaths, counting 1 to 4 on the in-breath and 1 to 8 on the out-breath while holding your attention on the breathing. Allow any tension to move out of your body as you slowly come to a more restful state.

Now shift your awareness to your mind. Is it quiet, or is it continuing to create thoughts, images, and feelings? A busy mind is always accompanied by tension in the body and a state of hyperactivity. The more inner noise is present, the more body tension you will have. Become aware of your body and notice how it feels with this specific level of mental activity. Give your current level of mental activity a number from one to ten, with one being a silent mind and ten the busiest mind you can imagine.

As your mental activity shifts, notice the corresponding shift in your body. Where is the tension in your body? Where do you mostly "hold" your tension? Most individuals have a particular spot, which can be indicated by a headache, stomach distress, bowel disturbances, or tight neck or back muscles. If you can locate such a spot it can serve as a biofeedback device, an early-warning sign of distress and imbalance. Both the level of your mental activity and the condition of your "tension spot" will inform you of an imbalance.

Return again to your breath. The breath is another subtle indicator of imbalance. Imagine yourself in a tense and difficult situation. Your breathing will be shallow, erratic, and it will predominantly use the chest muscles. Begin again to count your breaths as before: 1 to 4 on the in-breath and 1 to 8 on the out-breath. Notice how your body slows down and tension diminishes as your breath becomes regular and deeper, and makes use of your abdominal muscles. At any time during the day you can stop, observe your breath, and make a determination of the condition of your mind and body. The character of the breath and the level of mental activity move together so that each can serve as an early-warning device.

We have now looked at several "indicators" of body balance and imbalance. In addition to the *level* of mental activity, the *character* of this activity can also provide you with valuable information. Emotions such as confusion, boredom, anger, and anxiety all have a certain "energy" associated with them, a feeling of dis-ease and imbalance. It is important not to view these emotions as negative, something to be rid of, but rather as indicators of an inner imbalance. If one of these feelings is currently present, sit quietly with it and first notice where it is expressed in your body. If you can, intensify it so you are completely absorbed in this feeling.

Next follow this feeling back to other times in your life when you have had it. What were these circumstances? What are the patterns that relate them to your current situation? Are you experiencing disapproval, resentment, powerlessness, or helplessness? Where did you learn these feelings? Are there alternatives?

Next take your mind to a time in your life when you felt confident, strong, and in control. If you can't recall such a time, imagine one. Amplify these feelings until they fill your entire being. These are the feelings we spoke of earlier, the feelings of *hardiness* and *coherence.* For a moment, take these feelings into the circumstance that produced the distressing feelings. Are things different when your attitudes shift? Are your attitudes facilitating an inner calm, or healing?

In this exercise we have seen how the breath, body tension, your "tension spot," and negative emotions can serve as indicators of an inner imbalance. With this information, and using these experiences as guides, you can begin to make the changes that will allow for self-healing. When you are finished, review this exercise in your mind and then slowly open your eyes and return to the time and place of your surroundings.

᧬

The Homeostatic Healing System is our fundamental healing system. Without it we could never maintain the moment-to-moment checks and balances that are required to sustain life. But our consciousness and our capacity to create living conditions unimaginable to those who came before us now require us to understand and participate in its activities. Our role is to become aware at an early stage of the presence of imbalance and distress, symptoms that indicate that the homeostatic system has reached the limits of its adaptability. It is then time for us to use our resources and skills to reexamine our attitudes, lifestyles, relationships, and environments to determine which are to be adjusted in a manner that allows for the normal process of autoregulation and self-healing. In this way we can maximize the effectiveness of our natural healing mechanisms while minimizing the need for outside interventions, what we call treatment. In my view, we rarely require a theory, technique, practice, or practitioner to achieve inner balance. We already have a complete and intact system to do that for us.

FOUR

THE TREATMENT
HEALING SYSTEM

The machine does not isolate man from the great problems
of nature, but plunges him more deeply into them.
—Antoine de Saint-Exupéry

It is the folly of man that he believes and acts as if he can live
in ways and in environments that defy his nature. It is the
genius of man that has successfully devised a multitude of
treatment systems that respond to the pain and suffering associated with such violations and in part assist him in recovering
from his ill-considered confrontation with nature. Like ourselves, our ancestors could not avoid the necessary adversities
of living, but these adversities have escalated with modern
urban life, resulting in a myriad of toxic, stress-related, and
degenerative diseases of our own making.

As these diseases became more complex and prevalent, our
approaches to treatment became increasingly complex and essential to sustaining life. And, in our times, we have become
both creators and stewards of one of the most sophisticated
and elegant approaches to treatment ever known to man, biomedicine. In our ethnocentricity we often assume that this
uniquely Western expression of the scientific process is the

only credible treatment system. As we shall see, this is hardly the case.

Treatment is the use of an external remedy or practice for the purpose of assisting recovery from distress and disease. Humans have always sought methods of treatment. And these methods have differed from one culture to another. This explains the difference between the Homeostatic Healing System, a relatively fixed and universal system that is built into the body, and the great diversity of approaches that are contained within the framework of the Treatment Healing System. This system is a broad umbrella that allows for many different approaches to treatment, each sharing the common goal of repairing abnormalities and restoring normal function.

The host of treatment approaches that have evolved over the period of human existence contain a rich storehouse of information and possibilities. In order to draw from this large storehouse intelligently and effectively we must first appreciate the relative nature of any single approach; all approaches have something to offer us and no single one has a clear monopoly on either truth or efficacy. When it comes to treatment, each approach must step up to the plate and demonstrate its effectiveness.

Given this brief introduction to the Treatment Healing System, it becomes evident that biomedicine, acupuncture, chiropractic, Ayurvedic medicine, energy medicine, native and traditional medicine, homeopathy, and a host of other approaches usually fall under the umbrella of the Treatment Healing System. Each of these treatment approaches is based on a particular theory of health and disease. For example, Ayurveda proposes that the human body consists of three basic elements: Kapha, Pitta, and Vata. Disease is a result of the imbalance of these elements. The Ayurvedic practitioner would direct his or her diagnostic efforts at detecting this imbalance, and prescribe a therapeutic program that is aimed at correcting it through the use of various supplements and practices. The practices associated with the approaches mentioned

above range from drugs and surgery to needling and herbol-
ogy, spinal manipulation, Ayurvedic supplements, energy
transfer, natural supplements and traditional practices, and
homeopathic remedies.

When I place all of these practices under the treatment system I usually find that I have offended many practitioners who
consider their practices to be holistic and in no way compara-
ble to biomedicine. Here is an example of why I view these as
treatments. Ayurvedic healing derives from the much broader
approach to healing that we call Yoga. Yoga is not simply
about supplements and specific treatments, nor is it about
meditation used as a relaxation and stress-reduction technique. Yoga has eight branches, which, as a unit, direct themselves toward personal enlightenment—the expansion of
awareness and the experience of wholeness that is the essence
of healing. Taken together, the philosophy, theory, and practice of Yoga is beyond doubt a holistic approach to healing.
However, how many individuals who visit an Ayurvedic center
move beyond the treatments associated with this one aspect
of Yoga? How many individuals continue past their initial
exposure to Ayurveda, investing themselves in the long-term
effort of working with their minds and bodies to realize the
fundamental intention of this approach to healing? In my
view, when Ayurveda is separated from its place in the larger
frame of Yoga it becomes a treatment rather than a holistic
practice. The same can be said of the many other so-called
holistic therapies.

However holistic an approach may be in theory, when practiced in our culture, irrespective of the hype, it usually ends up
as a treatment that has largely lost its holistic origins. There is
an unfortunate but largely unavoidable tendency to carry our
extensive experience of the medical model into our search for
alternative treatments. In the process, we often medicalize and
reshape these approaches to conform to the overall architec-
ture of the medical model. We are so accustomed to thinking
in terms of the medical model that we rarely realize how this

conditioning follows us around. This is how we take a holistic approach such as Yoga and distill and reshape it until it becomes a narrow treatment approach, a way of fixing and repairing from the outside, new, but not new.

The tendency to "medicalize" or Westernize practices that are holistic in their orientation, or whose theories and practices are alien to biomedicine, can be seen clearly in the efforts of the "managed care" insurance programs to incorporate these practices into traditional insurance programs. Consider the case of acupuncture. Acupuncture is a specific practice that is an aspect of the much larger theory and practice of Chinese medicine, an approach that is comprehensive and holistic when taken in its entirety. When providing coverage for these services, insurance companies are choosing only to pay for the services that are directed at repairing a specific disorder. They can only "see" through the lens of the biomedical model. In the case of acupuncture, their coverage may be limited to the treatment of either chronic pain or addictive disorders. In this manner a theory and practice that is holistic is reduced to becoming another method of treating a specific disease. Its initial focus on the whole person is jettisoned and both the practitioner and the practice are corrupted.

Another trap we fall into is the belief that a practitioner has a holistic outlook merely because he or she uses multiple treatments. Although such a practitioner may well have a broader view of the *treatment possibilities*, his or her approach is often much of the same, using one or more practices to fix and repair an abnormality. Alternative practitioners often make use of a variety of terms such as "balancing the body" to suggest that their perspective is uniquely holistic. This changes nothing. Balancing the body through external manipulations is another form of treatment. It is important to evaluate what a practitioner is doing, not what he or she is saying. Holism is a perspective, a way we view life. It does not fix or repair, and no theory, practice, or practitioner can do it *to* you. It comes built in. It needs only to be recognized and experienced. It is a philosophy that emerges from and expresses the reality of our being.

BIOMEDICINE: ONE APPROACH TO TREATMENT

The discussion that follows can apply to any approach to treatment, but I have chosen to discuss biomedicine both because I am a practitioner of this approach and because it is the most prevalent method of treatment in this culture. Biomedicine is based on the principles we discussed in Chapter 2: objectivism, determinism, and positivism. In general, as a practitioner of biomedicine I believe that if we reduce our view to smaller and smaller sublevels of biology, with time research in biomedicine will discover a singular cause for every ailment. At its core, this belief ascribes the cause of disease to the dysfunction of our genes and basic physiology. If we can discover the unique and singular genetic or physiological abnormality we can then develop a "magic bullet" that will reverse the abnormality and its corresponding outward laboratory and physical markers. The primary practices associated with biomedicine are the use of drugs and surgery. As a practitioner, an expert in this system, my faith and approach are primarily invested in this perspective and its practices, which of course is as it should be.

Biomedicine, like other treatment systems, does not stand alone. It is supported by a large web of interconnected individuals and corporations, small and large, that are invested, through the profits from the sale of their goods and services, in the expansion of this system. The interests of this gigantic biomedical industry do not stem from its belief in the universal efficacy of this specific approach, but rather from its ongoing capacity to generate income. As a result, there can be a continued fueling and support of a specific approach regardless of an emerging recognition of its limitations. The final determination of the efficacy of an approach lies neither in the domain of those who are financially invested in it nor in practitioners whose perspectives are clouded by their training and obligatory allegiance to a specific approach.

The biomedical approach, like other treatment approaches, is administered by practitioners whose expertise conveys to them a sense of authority. This tends to relegate the patient to a more dependent position. For example, when patients enter my office they immediately become part of a culture with its designated roles, beliefs, rituals, and practices. This conditioned process is subtle, complex, and largely, given human nature, unavoidable. Even practitioners who ascribe to multiple approaches find themselves in the same situation, several times multiplied. How else can it be? Practitioners, by definition, have hopefully invested themselves in becoming experts in one particular area. This requires a focus that by necessity largely excludes other approaches.

If I look carefully at biomedicine, an act that for any practitioner is somewhat dangerous and undermining, I cannot but discover that as an approach to treatment, biomedicine is not universal in its efficacy, as I have been taught. There are areas in which it is highly effective—for example, acute trauma, surgical interventions, the treatment of bacterial infections, and preventive immunization—and areas in which it is highly ineffective—for example, stress-related disorders, degenerative and chronic diseases, and the promotion of high-level health. For an individual seeking assistance in resolving distress it is essential to understand the *range of effectiveness* of a specific approach before choosing it. How, you may ask, can I assess the range of effectiveness of a particular treatment approach? First you must find out what its capabilities are and, second, you must consider them in the context of other approaches to treatment.

For example, let's return to Ann's case, which we discussed in Chapter 1. After the diagnosis of cervical cancer she was offered the therapy favored by biomedicine—surgical removal of the tumor. But there were also other therapies for her to consider, including her final choice of a form of treatment that focused on supplements and a variety of alternative cancer drugs. What she failed to consider, and was most likely unaware of, was the range of effectiveness of each of these therapies. In her case, surgical removal of her cancer, the treatment promoted by biomedicine, has been documented to be highly effective for localized cervical cancer. The same could not be said with any level of assurance about the therapy she chose. Its range of effectiveness was either unknown or more in the area of opinion rather than documented fact. However, when considering the other aspects of her care, how best to support her mind and body through the surgical procedure and recovery process, and further, how to promote her long-term health, therapies outside of the biomedical model—approaches such as biofeedback, meditation, imagery, art and music therapy, Yoga, body work, and insight counseling, among others— would likely have a much broader range of effectiveness than any therapy found in the biomedical model.

Physicians, like other practitioners, exhibit a proficiency only in their particular approach. We cannot rely on them to provide us with a holistic and multidimensional view. That can only come from each of us. This is to say that *no practitioner can provide us with a full range of choices and options, and a knowledge of the range of effectiveness of specific alternative approaches.* The intelligent use of the treatment system therefore requires that *we* become holistic in our thinking, knowledgeable about the diversity of treatment approaches, and skillful in choosing among them. This is considerably more difficult than illogically jumping from one treatment approach to another. It calls for a growing maturity in the use of our healing capacities and the willingness to become as educated as we can about the varied approaches to treatment. As we will discuss later, innovations such as the Internet and its extensive on-line resources have the potential to provide us with quick access to the information we will each need. However, ultimately it will, and should, remain our responsibility to put all of that information together and make an educated and thoughtful decision. Ann's dilemma was not hers alone. It belongs to all of us. Living, as I have said earlier, in "in-between" times often leaves us with more information than we can deal with appropriately until we can find and use an organizing model.

GOOD INTENTIONS AND BAD RESULTS

The Treatment Healing System is the *only* one of the four healing systems that, in the routine use of its practices, generates a significant number of undesired and adverse side effects. *Iatrogenesis*, a term that comes from *iatro*, the Latin word for medicine, and *genesis*, the word meaning "coming from," refers to the undesired consequences that arise from the practice of any form of treatment, conventional or alternative. No approach to treatment is without its unique undesired effects.

There is a fragile balance between the sought-after reparative and restorative effects of a treatment approach and its disease-inducing effects. The more complex, technological, and sophisticated the approach (for example, biomedicine), the more extensive and serious are its adverse side effects. Similarly, the more dominance, authority, and exclusivity conveyed by a society to a specific approach, the more vulnerable that society becomes to the untoward effects of the practices associated with it. When choosing a treatment approach, the two major issues to consider are: the unwanted and usually unplanned physiological side effects, toxic and otherwise, and the more covert but perhaps even more significant psychosocial effects that are a direct result of the progressive medicalization of many aspects of our personal and social lives.

To look in our bathroom cabinets is to find numbers of labeled bottles that reflect, in a very personal way, the quantity of medications and supplements, prescribed and over-the-counter, that each of us consumes over the period of a year or more. As physicians and individuals we owe much thanks to computers that have given us a handle on the many interactions that occur among these drugs as they intermix in the mind and body. It is neither possible nor our intent to catalog the host of side effects, known and unknown, acute and chronic, that are associated with these therapies; there are other readily available sources that contain this information. For example, when it comes to biomedicine, *The Physician's Desk Reference* is an excellent resource that is now available at most bookstores. Unfortunately, it is far more difficult to access this information for other forms of treatment.

The fact is that regardless of all efforts to test and license these medications, what we don't know about them will always exceed what we do know. This same line of reasoning applies, more or less, to diagnostic testing, supplements, homeopathic remedies, herbs, manipulations, and the variety of practices associated with treatment. The more intensive and interventionist a practice or procedure is, the higher the potential for untoward side effects, both in number and seriousness. The fact is that whenever we choose to use therapeutic agents we take on the ever-present possibility of their side effects. To the extent that we find ourselves increasingly dependent on treatments, we will also find ourselves increasingly vulnerable to their unavoidable side effects. This is a built-in reality of treatment, whether conventional or alternative.

Perhaps of greater significance is the cost to us of a healing system that invariably leads to the loss of self-care skills, denies the presence of our inner healing capacities, discourages personal autonomy, and medicalizes the universal concerns with disease, pain and suffering, aging, and death. When we visit a practitioner and invest ourselves in a particular approach, we rarely consider these consequences, consequences that are a covert result of *all* approaches to treatment. They do not result from one visit, or perhaps even from a number of visits, but rather from the long-term, exclusive, and pervasive influence of the Treatment Healing System on a culture, an influence that is felt from cradle to grave.

Every time I prescribe a medication or another practitioner prescribes his or her form of treatment, we are toying with a very sharp knife that cuts two ways: In one direction it augments the process of recovery; in the opposite direction it cuts the individual off from his or her experience, denying the patient access to deeper intentions, personal growth and development, and, in fact, long-term potential for high-level health. For example Zantac reduces the acid in the stomach and thereby eliminates the pain associated with ulcers. However, it also relieves an individual of the motivation and uniquely human responsibility to explore the nature of his or her experience, the sources of distress, and its implications for life. Prozac may lift an individual from the darkness of a vegetative depression, enabling further growth and development; however it can also separate the person from the essential process of self-discovery and self-awareness that is motivated and fueled by the pain and suffering of depression. A coronary artery bypass procedure may eliminate angina and increase function, but it may also deny an individual the opportunity to take an essential look at the critical issues of midlife. I have used illustrations from biomedicine because it is our predominant healing tradition. But it is important to remember that these concerns are not unique to biomedicine; they are found in all approaches to treatment, conventional and alternative. The Treatment Healing System, when used exclusively, is at all times a potential threat to personal autonomy and to the development of full health.

Life has never been and will never be without its existential problems. Disease, aging, pain and suffering, and death are inseparable from the human condition. At their core they are highly personal issues, and over a lifetime we must each confront and cope with them. How convenient it has become to rid ourselves of these unpleasant aspects of life by turning them over to be repaired by a waiting professional or institution. To the extent that we are separated from these essential aspects of living by the medicalization and psychologizing of the core elements of the human condition, our health and autonomy, in Ivan Illich's words, are expropriated by professionals, institutions, and belief systems. Whether and how we take on these life issues determines the quality and extent of our experience. To turn them over to others is to deny fundamental aspects of our lives.

I am increasingly aware that it may be more important for us to assume responsibility for the psychosocial and spiritual aspects of healing, to expand our consciousness and self-reliance, and to extend our capacities and resources than it may be to replace one treatment approach with another. I do not mean to suggest that we should cease our exploration of alternative treatments, but rather that we reconsider our priorities and broaden our perspectives.

NAVIGATING THE TREATMENT HEALING SYSTEM

Of the four healing systems, the treatment system is undoubtedly the most difficult to navigate, particularly in our time when aspects of biomedicine are called into doubt, and when we are confronted with many different treatment approaches, some old and some new, some effective and others not. Several guidelines are important:

• No one treatment system has all the answers.

• The treatment healing system is only one of four healing systems, each of which should be considered when designing a healing program.

- Practitioners are most devoted to and knowledgeable about the specifics of their particular approach.

- Every treatment approach has both benefits and risks, and, as we have discussed, the risks are both direct and indirect.

- Choosing to use a treatment system is a two-level decision. First, given the four healing systems, which is the best option? Second, what is the most appropriate treatment approach within that system?

- There is no substitute for your own research. Consider the following questions:
    What is the theory behind this approach?
    What is its track record for my particular problem?
    Where can I get this information?
    Does this approach consider the other healing systems?
    Is the practitioner well trained and broad in his or her outlook?

- The older and more established healing traditions, for example, traditional Chinese healing, Ayurveda, homeopathy, and chiropractic, provide more depth and reassurance than newer and untested approaches.

- When choosing a practitioner, check out his or her credentials, and then "feel out" his or her heart. They are both essential. Consider the following questions:
    Does the practitioner converge in on a symptom or diagnosis quickly, without asking about what else is happening in the rest of your life?
    Does he or she insist there is only one effective approach? Although this may be so, at the least a combination of approaches addressing mind, body, and spirit is a more effective way to go.
    Does the practitioner offer you time to consider the options he or she proposes?
    Does the practitioner *ever* consider options outside of his or her area of expertise?

> Are you comfortable with this person?
> Does he or she seem happy, relaxed, and at peace?

• Take your time and consider your choices carefully.

It must be quite apparent by now that more information is needed to evaluate the different treatment approaches and their efficacy with specific problems. This is slowly occurring through research such as that funded by the Office of Alternative Medicine at the National Institutes of Health. Ongoing efforts to provide reliable information also include the development of peer-reviewed journals that publish research regarding alternative treatment approaches, and the increasing availability of newsletters for the general public. It is my view, expressed throughout this book, that the development of the information superhighway will in time provide each of us with all the information we need, a process that will surely begin the collapse of the distinction between professional and layperson, liberating us to become orchestrators of our own health and healing. As explorers in this new world of healing, we must accustom ourselves to slow and thoughtful steps as we move toward our final goal of a diverse and fully integrated healing system.

∽

INNER JOURNEY #4: MANAGING TREATMENT

Find a comfortable place to sit and allow thirty minutes for this exercise.

Begin by closing your eyes and shifting into a more silent inner state, letting go of all thoughts and activities. Imagine that over the past year you have been suffering from recurrent headaches that have no cause that is apparent to you. After exhausting all that you can do, what is your next recourse? (Consider your choices.)

If you need help, you will likely call upon a helper, a practitioner of one sort or another. In our tradition this would likely be a physician. Place yourself in this individual's office. How does it feel? Do you feel empowered or disempowered? What are you asking for? What are the words you use? What will you be satisfied with? Spend some time, before the practitioner enters, considering the expectations you bring to this encounter, your strengths and your vulnerabilities.

Next observe your encounter with the practitioner. What are your feelings? What are your respective roles? What is the range of possibilities that exist in this encounter, the possible interventions? Is the dialogue directed solely toward repair and rehabilitation? Is this satisfying to you? How much do you know about the efficacy of this approach? Will you be satisfied that you have accomplished your goals if the headache is eradicated? Follow this encounter to its end, observing its intention and its outcome.

Now let's return home and begin again, this time in front of your computer. Turn it on and imagine you know how to retrieve information from the Internet. Call up all information regarding headaches, particularly the information that pertains to your type of headache. Read through the different treatment approaches, their efficacy and side effects.

Next enter your personal data into the computer and call up the case histories of others who have shared your precise problem. This may require that you first complete a computer-based personal history and symptom-based questionnaire. Examine the case histories, the approaches used, and the outcomes. Perhaps you may want to E-mail one of the individuals responding, or further evaluate a treatment approach by reading through the supporting research. Or perhaps you want to speak through E-mail to an expert in this field.

When you have completed this process, plan your treatment. If this involves a practitioner, imagine yourself in his or her office. How do you feel now, empowered or disempowered? What is the character of your interaction? Beyond the specific result of any specific treatment, what have you learned? Was the healing more about a treatment, or about the knowledge you gained about yourself, your capacities, or the deeper sources of the headache?

When you have completed the exercise, open your eyes and return to the time and space of your surroundings.

∾

I hope that this exercise has given you a firsthand sense of the capacities and resources that are increasingly available to you as you begin to orchestrate your own health and healing. How you approach it makes all the difference. As you explore these issues in the following chapters, I think you will agree that we must expand the conversation from one that exclusively focuses on substituting one treatment approach for another to a larger conversation that includes consideration of the other healing systems, accompanied by the expansion of our personal skills, resources, and knowledge.

CONSCIOUSNESS: THE ACTIVATING FACTOR

The hero-deed to be wrought today is not what it was in the century of Galileo. Where there was darkness, now there is light; where light was, now there is darkness. The modern hero-deed must be that of questing to bring to light again the lost Atlantis of the co-ordinated soul.

—Joseph Campbell

In our discussion of the four healing systems we have now arrived at a place that is identical to the place where I invariably arrive when caring for individuals in my medical practice. Consider the following cases: Susan, a thirty-eight-year-old professional working seventy hours a week in a high-stress job while recovering from an ulcer; Steve, twenty-four years old, who is suffering from colitis; Howard, in his mid-fifties, undergoing rehabilitation from his first heart attack; and Marilyn, a forty-year-old mother of three children suffering from recurrent headaches. In each instance we can either move forward and activate the Mind/Body and Spiritual Healing Systems, or satisfy ourselves with the partial and often temporary relief provided by the treatment system.

I would like to tell you that Susan, Steve, Howard, and Marilyn grasped at the opportunity to move toward Whole Healing, but I can't. Because we have grown accustomed to the treatment system, its professionals and techniques, there is a strong resistance to taking the initiative and making the effort to develop the inner resources and capacities required for mind/body and spiritual healing, and as a result, change comes slowly. Whole Healing requires a choice, an intentional choice to expand our consciousness and explore the depths of our being. But more than a change in consciousness must occur; a change in consciousness accompanied by a change in how we see ourselves and our possibilities, a shift in our worldview, must take place. When we make this choice, we activate the Mind/Body and Spiritual Healing Systems, setting into motion and energizing the Whole Healing System. Looking back on my twenty-five years of medical practice, I am certain that more than ever before we all want to be a part of a dynamic and participatory healing process, one that moves beyond partial healing.

I saw an example of this several years ago when I visited with a group of individuals who, under the supervision of Dr. Dean Ornish, had chosen a new approach to working with coronary heart disease, a disease that had significantly disabled their lives. Each participant had used the treatment system and its resources—drugs, coronary bypass surgery, and angioplasty—to heal their disease. Then Dr. Ornish offered them a further possibility: the use of the Mind/Body and Spiritual Healing Systems.

In Ornish's study, which at the time of my visit had been underway for a period of four years, participants were directly involved in their healing: They learned the effects of different foods on their illness and changed their diets dramatically, they practiced Yoga and meditation, began regular exercise routines, and met in small groups to discuss the program and their lives. During the study, intermittent testing of the participants indicated that seemingly permanent and expanding coronary obstructions were, as a direct result of changes in attitudes, activities, and nutritional practices, partially reversing themselves—reversing themselves without the use of drugs.

In the course of my visit I was inspired not so much by the change in the condition of the participants' coronary vessels, but by what I understood as their change in consciousness and worldview. The individuals I met were beaming with vitality, energy, and enthusiasm. They had added the Mind/ Body and Spiritual Healing Systems to their original approach and by so doing had initiated themselves into very different lives. The pivotal shift was the expansion of consciousness, the essential ingredient that activated the Mind/Body and Spiritual Healing Systems. Their disease had helped them to discover the essence of whole health: using the complete healing system.

THE STRUCTURE OF CONSCIOUSNESS

Because of its pivotal role in Whole Healing, it is important that we pause to explore the act of consciousness as it applies to each of the four healing systems. Consciousness operates differently in each of these systems. With homeostasis, consciousness is inborn and acts automatically as built-in instinct. With treatment, consciousness is reactive, responding to distress according to culturally imposed perspectives (in our culture the biomedical system). With mind/body healing, consciousness changes profoundly; it is intentional and deliberately activated. And with spiritual healing, consciousness is intuitive, capable of grasping the deeper patterns and relationships that are found in wholeness. Unlike the homeostatic and treatment systems, which are primarily reactive, restoring balance only when it is lost, intentional and spiritual consciousness are oriented toward the long-term achievement of Whole Healing and full health, an orientation that is well demonstrated by Dr. Ornish's patients.

The Role of Consciousness in Whole Healing

Healing System	Homeostasis	Treatment	Mind/Body	Spiritual
Aspect of Consciousness	Instinctual	Reactive	Intentional	Intuitive

Each of the four healing systems is distinguished by a different aspect of consciousness. Instinctual consciousness is given at birth, reactive consciousness is shaped by our past experiences, and intentional and intuitive consciousness are proactively developed as a result of personal choice and effort. Intentional and intuitive consciousness allow for the expansion of our healing capacities.

When we consider the role of consciousness, as depicted above, it is helpful to view the four aspects of consciousness as different TV channels, each with its own characteristics. We usually run on Channels 1 and 2, instinctive and reactive consciousness. As we become more self-directed, we add Channel 3, and if we continue in these efforts we will finally tune in to Channel 4, intuitive consciousness. In the undeveloped mind, the channel selector always reverts to Channel 1, which automatically maintains the basic functions of the mind and body, and Channel 2, which automatically directs our thoughts and actions through the conditioning of our preexisting, culturally based perspectives. Although many individuals can live an entire lifetime predominantly using Channels 1 and 2, others develop, to a more or less extent, the further capacities of the mind. The development of these capacities is the essential factor in the unfolding of the complete healing system. Jung describes this shift from automatic and reactive processing to intentional and intuitive awareness:

> The difference between the "natural" individuation process, which runs its course unconsciously, and the one which is consciously realized, is tremendous. In the first case consciousness nowhere intervenes; the end remains as dark as the beginning. In the second case so much darkness comes to light that the personality is permeated with light, and consciousness necessarily gains in scope and insight.

INSTINCTUAL CONSCIOUSNESS

Instinctual consciousness begins at conception. Coded into the fertilized egg is the pattern for the development of the whole, the fully realized human. Part of this initial patterning is the array of physiological checks and balances that automatically assures survival by responding to environmental stress and strain on our bodies in a manner that returns our physiology to a normal, steady state. Although the basic requirements of life contain some flexibility such as the permissible range of blood sugar, minerals, hormone levels, core temperature, and so on, there are strict limits to how far we can deviate from our basic life needs without threatening survival. The body has a way of knowing, a sort of consciousness, that both remembers the appropriate balances and can instinctually activate itself to reset these balances when they are threatened.

The homeostatic process is dependent on this internal feedback that informs it about the state of the system and the capacity to initiate the appropriate response. I have called this automatic and unconscious awareness and responsiveness *instinctual* consciousness. We are not accustomed to thinking of consciousness in this manner. When we think about consciousness we usually think of intelligence, memory, and decision making. But when we look carefully, we discover that a certain kind of consciousness is built into the body's automatic balancing systems. The noted physician Walter Cannon first referred to and described this type of intelligence in his book *The Wisdom of the Body*. I have always felt that these words, "the wisdom of the body," beautifully express the character and nature of instinctual consciousness.

REACTIVE CONSCIOUSNESS

We are initiated into reactive consciousness by our parents, teachers, and culture. It slowly builds as we collect factual and psychological information from our life experiences. This information is arranged and stored as ideas and concepts that rigidly define and guide our interpretations and responses to the events of our lives. Reactive consciousness often contains false information that is inadvertently acquired from others early in life, or partial information that is absorbed from those who have not as yet fully developed their own understanding. Until our consciousness is more fully developed we act upon this information as if it were accurate and complete.

This aspect of consciousness functions like a rapid automatic-response unit, quickly evaluating new information within the context of our preexisting perspectives and then reacting from a well-developed and predetermined set of responses. Reactive consciousness is linked to and always reflects information acquired in the past. It is based on an automatic judgment followed by an automatic response. Judgments are our personal "takes" on a specific event, requiring us to dip into our memories of past experiences. I am not suggesting that reactive consciousness, because it is linked to the past, is necessarily dysfunctional or inappropriate (consider how we learned to get out of the way of a moving car immediately), but rather that it lacks creativity. Instead, it promotes and defends preexisting ideas, perspectives, and behaviors—even when they no longer meet our present-day needs. It does, however, offer a consistency to our experience, weaving the same patterns, for good or for bad, throughout our lives. The price for this consistency is true creativity, vitality, and whole health.

For an example of our automatic and reactive responses, consider how we are guided by the narrow framework of the treatment system. We learn about the elements of this system early in life: the role of the professional and patient, the ticket of admission to the system (symptoms such as pain, bleeding, or the appearance of a new lump), the treatment methods and their "effectiveness." We also learn the system's values: an emphasis on parts rather than the whole, repair rather than integration, physicalness, "scientific proof," and unquestioning compliance. As we inherit this information it is carefully programmed into our minds, providing us with a consistent and predictable automated approach to the distress in our lives. At times this approach is highly effective in resolving our problems (for example, quickly calling 911 and going to the emergency ward after severe trauma), but quite often it is not (for example, using the biomedical model as the exclusive approach to the complex disorders of modern life). Because of our programming, even when reactive consciousness is inappropriate and ineffective we continue to believe in and use it.

INTENTIONAL CONSCIOUSNESS

Intentional consciousness develops through the disillusionments, failures, and wounds of our lives. We don't easily give up our automatic and accustomed ways of being. We do so only when we are forced to find a better way. The basic ingredient of intentional consciousness is a present-moment awareness that breaks through our preexisting perspectives and allows us to see the world and our experiences as they actually are rather than as we "color" them by past experience. Intentional consciousness pays attention to what is happening in our lives rather than to the endless internal dialogue of old thoughts, feelings, and images. It allows us to make choices based on what is right for a particular circumstance rather than automatically relying on old patterns and ways of doing things. The capacity for real choice allows for new initiatives, one of which is to expand what we have been taught about the treatment system to include an exploration of the potential of the Mind/Body and Spiritual Healing Systems.

One way to understand intentional consciousness is to consider an example from your own life, perhaps an attempt to change your diet, initiate an exercise program, or alter a form of behavior. When you forget your new intention you switch back to reactive consciousness, returning to Channel 2. The response is so automatic that when it occurs it is unlikely you will notice it. As you become aware that you are "doing the same old thing," you can consciously choose to reassert your desired new behavior. This is the shift to intentional consciousness. You can watch this shifting back and forth throughout the day. When you become numb to your current choices and become lost in old thought patterns, you have reverted to reactive consciousness. In a sense it is quite simple—intentional consciousness is being aware of what you are doing when you're doing it. It is psychological freedom.

INTUITIVE CONSCIOUSNESS

The fourth aspect of consciousness, intuitive consciousness (or we could equally say spiritual consciousness) provides for a knowledge that is very different from the knowledge gained exclusively through an objective science. One can experience it naturally, or be led to it through an expanding awareness. It is separate from our intellect or psychology, and though it isn't based on the accumulation of facts as information, there is a definitive certainty to it. Intuitive consciousness is neither contained nor influenced by any system of thoughts or beliefs. *It is the capacity to see below the surface of things, to apprehend patterns, relationships, and hidden meanings.*

Because it is poorly conveyed by words, intuitive consciousness can only be personally experienced, or intimated, through art, poetry, music, or symbol. It is a particular way of experiencing and sensing the essential intangibilities of life that is quite personal. At the same time, because it intuits larger patterns and relationships, it is quite impersonal. In the poem "Tintern Abbey," William Wordsworth beautifully describes intuitive consciousness as "a sense sublime / Of something far more deeply interfused."

Intuitive consciousness does not provide us with what we would consider to be practical information. It is not pragmatic in the usual sense. Rather, it provides us with wisdom, with a way to comprehend and organize the diverse experiences of life, the joys and pains, the gains and losses, successes and failures, and the great transitions of birth, aging, and death. It is not a substitute for the other aspects of consciousness, but rather an essential complement. It provides us with a transcendent overview of life that activates the soul and spirit, bringing vitality, peace, and sweetness to life.

As we expand our consciousness, we increasingly accumulate islands of larger awareness, which, with time, congeal into even larger "land masses." Because expanding consciousness takes time, we must be patient.

I have learned to appreciate the fact that consciousness unfolds in each of us according to our unique rhythm, pace, and style. The capacity to unveil and use the complete healing system, a capacity gained through the expansion of consciousness, is always present, but apparently it is not accessible to all people at all times. Nature has its reasons, a fact I now accept rather than question. We do not need to visit a monastery or an ashram to expand our consciousness. Instead, the routine activities of daily life, our relationships, work, and what we often believe to be mundane experiences can stimulate the full expansion of consciousness, an act that allows for the full activation of mind/body and spiritual healing.

SIX

THE MIND/BODY
HEALING SYSTEM

Aesthetic or intellectual flirtations with life or fate come to an abrupt halt here: the step to higher consciousness leaves us without a rear guard and without shelter. The individual must devote himself to the way with all his energy, for it is only by means of his integrity that he can go further, and his integrity alone can guarantee that his way will not turn out to be an absurd misadventure.

C. G. Jung

The initiation into an expanded consciousness, and the accompanying shift toward a self-directed life, are essential elements of mind/body healing. The Mind/Body Healing System is present at birth. However, it remains dormant until *we* choose to develop it. That is, nature provides us with a flexible and adaptive means to healing, one that is under our control. But unlike homeostasis and treatment, mind/body healing relies entirely on inner resources. It is proactive and intentional, and shifts the focus of healing toward the promotion of long-term well being.

Two components are essential to mind/body healing: *self-regulation* and *self-exploration*. Self-regulation is the capacity to intentionally direct and manage the operations of our minds and bodies, a capacity that can help us to recover from illnesses and promote health. Self-exploration is the process of examining the breadth and depth of our lives, a process that, over a lifetime, can diminish our inner conflicts and lead to the development of attitudes and perspectives consistent with health.

It is important to note that some current practitioners of mind/body healing gravely misunderstand its intent and direction. They see it as another form of treatment, a way of summoning the resources of the mind and body to accomplish what previously was the domain of the treatment system. This may be a step in the right direction, but if this is all we have achieved, we will have substituted one approach that seeks to repair and manipulate the body with another, albeit one that is self-directed and self-initiated. The true focus of the Mind/Body Healing System is on inner development, the mastery of new resources and skills, the expansion of consciousness, and the movement toward self-reliance. To fail to understand this distinction is to forfeit the benefits of Whole Healing.

SELF-REGULATION

Not long ago scientists believed that few, if any, of the workings of the mind and body were amenable to self-regulation. This is no longer the case. Johanna Schults, a psychiatrist and neurologist, first demonstrated in the early 1900s how individuals, through a series of self-instructions, were capable of inducing muscle relaxation, changing blood-pressure levels, varying the pulse rate, and causing the temperature of skin to rise or fall. Elmer and Alyce Green of the Menninger Clinic, pioneers in the development of biofeedback, extended these findings. Through the use of electronic feedback devices they trained individuals to fine-tune their ability to regulate body functions. Herbert Benson, a research physician at Harvard, further demonstrated how a technique as simple as meditation could result in predictable physiological changes throughout the body. Finally, Robert Ader, the scientist who initiated the field of psychoneuroimmunology, discovered that the immune system, our natural defense mechanism, was subject to intentional control. We now know that we have the capacity to regulate, to one degree or another, most of the activities of our minds and bodies. It has taken centuries, but we are finally learning to accept what ancient Yogis have always known.

Learning self-regulation requires determination and effort. Yet self-regulation can be as simple as choosing to spend time alone when the mind and body are overactive and need rest, taking time off from work to recover from illness, scheduling vacations rather than accumulating sick time, and as we shall shortly see, developing healthy and sustaining relationships. In fact, I often find myself encouraging patients to do these very things, but for many individuals these are not necessarily minor adjustments. When what would seem obvious is ignored, the result can be a delayed recovery from illness, and an increased susceptibility to disease. It is ironic that with all my years of professional training the most expert advice I give is often related to self-regulation, and that is "Take care of yourself." Patients often comply if I write a prescription for a medication, arrange for physical therapy, or suggest another medical treatment. Unfortunately, when it comes to self-regulation, they usually find it dispensable. I am getting in the habit of writing advice for self-regulation on a prescription pad: *Take two days off to rest from your viral infection.* When I do this my patients sometimes laugh. These moments show why mind/body healing is intentional rather than automatic. It cannot be prescribed; it must be chosen.

Self-regulation can be accomplished in a number of ways. The practices include meditation, Yoga, biofeedback, imagery, exercise, and nutrition. When these practices are combined they can work synergistically to contribute to recovery from a variety of ailments. For example, they can help control high blood pressure, prevent or reduce the effects of migraine headaches, reverse the lesions of heart disease, regulate hormone levels, normalize abnormal bowel motility, control cardiac arrythmias, and potentially influence the operations of the immune system.

Consider once more Dr. Ornish's patients, individuals with severe heart disease. They followed a simple program, but with profound results. Using exercise, Ornish's patients improved the efficiency of their cardiovascular systems, stabilized blood-sugar levels, increased muscle strength, and improved their sense of well-being. Through dietary modification, particularly by dramatically lowering cholesterol intake and increasing the intake of carbohydrates, they significantly reduced blood sugar and cholesterol levels, and diminished their susceptibility to a variety of cancers that are in part related to dietary fat levels. Using meditation and Yoga, they increased muscle suppleness and flexibility, reduced blood pressure, altered the stress-related overstimulation of hormonal-based systems, enhanced the effectiveness of the immune system, and simultaneously regulated any number of secondary processes. They were using self-regulation to alter the course of their disease.

How could Marie, whom we saw earlier, have used the Mind/Body Healing System, particularly self-regulation, for her asthma? Marie recognized her breathing problem only when it was overtly symptomatic, that is, she was unable to identify the subtle changes that preceded the dramatic symptoms. Self-regulation, like other therapies, is most effective at the earliest stages of a disorder, so I would have first discussed with her the idea of registering for a Yoga course to develop a greater sensitivity to her mind, body, and breathing. Yoga would also assist her in learning the most effective way to breathe, a basic skill for asthmatics. She would discover as well the difference between the feeling of complete relaxation and the feeling of a mere lowering of stress levels, something that each of us can discover for ourselves.

The second activity I would have suggested to Marie is biofeedback training. This self-regulation training process would have enabled her to prevent, diminish, or reverse the bronchospasms (the contraction of the muscles surrounding the breathing tubes) that are the most immediate cause of her symptom of breathlessness. Because the idea of the mind/body connection was somewhat new to her, she would do better learning these skills with the assistance of a formal teaching process rather than the less structured approach of meditation. To these activities I would have added moderate exercise, accompanied by a healthy diet. Further, I would have discussed with Marie some of the simple approaches mentioned above: finding the proper balance between work and play, scheduling time alone, and expanding her supportive relationships. As you can see, this would have required a rather profound shift in Marie's thinking, requiring her to stop merely depending on professionals and their therapies and to start depending on Marie and her own healing capacities. She would have had to move from a singular idea of causation (remember her statement, "It's the pollen, I know it") to the idea that illness is the result of a complex web of circumstances that can be approached from many directions at the same time.

For Marie, these two approaches to self-regulation, Yoga and biofeedback, would result in an expansion of awareness, and many fruitful discussions that would touch upon the process of Whole Healing. At a later time, when we would be well along with these initial activities, I would begin to discuss with her another aspect of self-regulation, one that recognizes that self-regulation is not limited to inner processes like biofeedback and meditation.

As social beings our involvement with the outer world also affects our health, and the principles of self-regulation extend to our interactions with other people, places, and things. For example, we can profoundly influence our health and healing by organizing and directing the character and extent of our social relationships.

There is considerable scientific evidence that supports the important link between relationships and health. For example, in 1979 researchers Lisa F. Berkman and S. Leonard Syme reported on a survey that measured the levels of social support of 6,928 adults in Alameda County, California. They considered the following four types of relationships: marriage, contacts with close friends and relatives, church membership, and informal and formal group associations. Nine years later, they examined the death rates in this same group of people. Their findings demonstrated that individuals who lacked social support and community ties were more likely to die during the nine-year follow-up period than those with more extensive contacts. In fact, they were 2½ times more likely to die. This result was *independent* of initial health status, socioeconomic status, health practices (smoking, alcoholic beverage consumption, physical activity, obesity, and use of health services). Similar studies in other communities and other cultures have shown much the same result. The implications are clear: When it comes to relationships and health, the more the better.

There is more to this story. Other studies have confirmed what many of us have discovered for ourselves: Following the death of a loved one, an intimate partner is at a higher risk for the development of unexpected disease and death, a risk that extends throughout the period of grieving. All of us who have suffered the loss of an important relationship are aware of how this can affect our health. Just as loss could have an impact on health, ongoing unhealthy relationships demonstrate a similar, although less drastic effect on health. Add to these the observation by David Spiegel, a psychiatrist and clinical researcher, that social support in the form of group psychotherapy may prolong survival in breast-cancer patients. Dr. Spiegel, using his skills as a psychiatrist, established a support group for those patients, and the result, unexpected by Dr. Spiegel, showed that the women in the support group lived twice as long as a similar group of patients who did not participate in such a group.

The question these studies raise is, How does the well-being we feel when we are properly supported in relationship affect our physical state? Does feeling good emotionally change the way our molecules behave? We have already seen in the work of Antonovsky and Kobassa that the ability to resist the effects of stress and adversity were directly related to certain personal qualities (resourcefulness, managcability, meaningfulness, inner control, a positive outlook, and a sturdy sense of self), qualities that, we are discovering through research in psychoneuroimmunolgy, affect our biochemistry and therefore our health. Our systems of social support enhance the development of these qualities.

In light of these findings it is fair next to ask, *How* do our relationships support and encourage these qualities? Family, friends, and other acquaintances provide us with helpful and practical information, give us support at times of need, encourage healthy behavior, and serve as a "mirror" in which we can see ourselves, both what we like and what we don't like. They also provide us with companionship, warmth, affection, and the assurance of physical touch (we all know how important touch is, but rarely give thought to how it may actually influence our physiology and psychology). The special relationship we call intimacy is an important way to meet the essential human need to bond to others. The healthy connectedness that is possible between people, as opposed to dysfunctional dependent relationships, helps us to grow, develop, and mature in our lives.

Consider our current circumstance. Historically, most humans spend a lifetime receiving support from 50 to 150 steady and reliable individuals. In our time, each year, 20 percent of the population relocates, half every 5 years. The average household has dropped from 4.1 members in 1930 to 2.8 members in 1980, and 42 percent of households include only one person. In the process of these social changes, we have created a new and very significant risk factor for disease and premature death: social isolation. When we do not have the supportive and warm relationships essential for health, we have limited our capacity for Whole Healing.

The implications for self-regulation are clear: First we need to learn how to choose, create, and sustain healthy relationships, and then we need to expand our circle of relationships. The skills that are required for healthy relationships, such as communication, conflict resolution, and listening skills, are not taught in school, nor do many of us have the opportunity to observe them at work in our families. The alternative, learning by trial and error, is both time consuming and often needlessly destructive. There are now many good books, seminars, and counselors who can help individuals develop this aspect of their self-regulatory capacity. Relationship is, like the other self-regulatory practices, a learned skill, one that we must choose and pursue if we wish to develop the Mind/Body Healing System. From my discussions with patients, I am certain that developing the skills that would help them expand and enhance their relationships would be a significant aspect of an effective mind/body approach to their illnesses.

SELF-EXPLORATION

The second aspect of mind/body healing is self-exploration. Unlike self-regulation, a skill that can be immediately applied to directing and managing the operations of the mind and body, self-exploration is more subtle. When pursued, it results in a more complete understanding of ourselves, an understanding that is not limited to an awareness of our day-to-day thoughts and feelings, but extends into the recesses of our minds, enabling us to understand our fears, anxieties, emotions, hopes, dreams, special talents, and unique temperament. The result is a more harmonious and authentic life, one that comes to terms with our past and informs us how to live in the present in a way that is consistent with who and what we are. And we may well discover that this is in sharp contrast to what

we may perhaps have become, often as a result of the unhealthy influence of well-meaning others.

I am reminded of a short vignette related by Joseph
Campbell at a workshop I attended. He told the story of a
man who spent his entire life climbing a ladder until he finally reached the top rung. As he looked over the top, he discovered that he had placed his ladder against the wrong wall
and what he thought was there, was not. For all of his efforts, he now had to come down the ladder, and find the
right wall. Thus the important effort, he discovered, was not
in the climbing, but in knowing in the beginning how to recognize the right wall.

Self-exploration gives us the information we need to find
the right wall. If we follow, consciously or unconsciously, the
inherited advice of our culture or our loved ones, we may
make incorrect choices. However tedious acquiring self-
knowledge may seem at times, if we know enough about ourselves we do not end up disappointed, angry, resentful, or
finger-pointing. We live our *own* lives. And it is when we live
according to our unique nature that our minds, bodies, and
spirits are integrated and balanced. This is the form of healing
that results from the commitment to self-exploration.

Most of us are not up to the task of effective self-exploration.
Our minds, with their constant inner chatter, persist in re-
analyzing the same information repeatedly and invariably
come up with the same answers, answers that work no better
upon reexamination than the first time they were tried. To understand ourselves, our lives, or the world around us we must
experience them without preconceived notions, biases, prejudices, or any other perspectives that will stop us from living
each experience with clarity, freshness, and originality. *As we
pursue the process of self-exploration, the first step is the capacity to induce and sustain inner silence. The second step is
learning and using a series of skills of self-inquiry that can
help us get the information we need, information that we are
usually unaware of.*

SILENCING THE MIND

Silencing the mind can be initiated through meditation or relaxation techniques, Yoga practices, breathing exercises, time spent in nature, through music, dance, and a host of other activities. Each of us can find what works best for us; in fact, we may already know. Silence, however, is not an easy skill to develop and use. We often feel guilty about taking time for ourselves, particularly when it seems that we are subtracting it from time spent with family, loved ones, or work. We feel unproductive and selfish. We may also avoid silence because when we slow down we may experience thoughts and feelings that we have been avoiding by keeping busy. Finally, it comes down to an issue of values. If we wish to avoid silence it is quite easy to do so. However, if we value an in-depth understanding of ourselves, the discovery of new possibilities, and the activation of mind/body healing, we must recognize that this potential is discovered in silence.

Silence is the space between thoughts. Thoughts come from memory and reflect the experiences that are stored there. A thought is therefore tied to our particular life experiences and, as a result, to time. The silent space, a specific aspect of consciousness, is unrelated to memory. It does not contain thoughts and, as a result, it is unrelated to our past experiences. Silence is timeless, formless, infinite, and above all, thoughtless. It is a multipotential state with undefined and, in a sense, limitless possibilities. When the silence is broken by another thought, the thought will most likely be related to our past experiences. However, this is not how it must be. It is possible to "use" the space of silence, particularly when it is extended, in creative ways. Silence allows us to penetrate the surface layer of experience to perceive patterns and relationships, to discover new insights and understandings, and to experience wholeness and oneness.

We can only explore these possibilities if we are able to move beyond the day-to-day thoughts that occupy our minds.

These thoughts do not allow self-exploration. They only allow the continuous reanalysis of the same thought patterns. Because the untrained mind will always default back to its internal chatter, it is important for us to learn techniques that can both assist with inducing and sustaining silence, and then further assist us in using the silence to generate the insights and understandings we have talked about. You can begin with Inner Journey #5 later in this chapter, "Accessing Inner Silence." It shows you a meditation technique that, when regularly practiced, will help you learn how to silence your mind.

Silence is a very fragile commodity. Frequently, and without our awareness, it will give way to the distractions of a restless mind. We easily recognize its ephemeral quality when we return from a vacation, retreat, or meditation and resume our daily routines. When we first try it, we have difficulty with our capacity to still the mind. The most minimal stimulation can break our attention and reactivate our inner dialogues. For many years, these inner conversations have dominated our minds. To overcome their "long-term advantage" we must set aside a few moments each day to check the mind's noise level, and if necessary, to stop and quiet down. You can accomplish this by using your routine activities as an opportunity to practice this skill. Stop for a moment, pause, slow down, take five deep breaths, and feel the inner quiet. In this simple manner, all of us, regardless of the demands of our daily lives, can learn to quiet down quickly.

Once we become proficient in quieting our minds we may find it easy to get lost in the pleasure and peace of stillness. But pleasure and peace achieved in this way are as ephemeral as silence itself. They are not the goal of this aspect of mind/body healing—self-exploration is. It is at this point that many individuals stop their self-exploration. Instead they use meditation and other such activities as relaxation techniques, welcome interludes from an otherwise hectic day. For them, limiting their exposure to these practices is just another way to avoid living life, like another drink, pill, or dependent relationship. They constantly return to them, using these practices as a treatment to avoid, if only for the moment, the anxiety, pain, and suffering invariably associated with the unexamined life. They will never discover the "gold" that lies beneath the surface, because it does not reside exclusively in the silence, but rather in using the silence as a means to further self-exploration and mind/body healing.

SELF-INQUIRY

You can develop specific skills that can assist you in learning more about yourself. As mentioned earlier, these are not day-to-day problem-solving skills, but rather self-inquiry skills that can help you to go below the surface of your experience to gather information that is usually hidden from your view. In the sections below I suggest four practices I regularly use with my patients, practices that can enhance your capacity for self-inquiry. Read them through and practice one at a time, finding the practice or practices that are most helpful for you. As you work with them you may develop variations on these practices that specifically fit your style.

The first approach works automatically, relying on your mind's capacity, when it is silent, to generate creative insights spontaneously. Once your mind is silent, the thoughts, feelings, and images that create your usual mental chatter are, for the moment, gone. This allows the mind to activate your imagination, much as it does during the silence of sleep. Like your dreams, your imagination contains information not obvious to your day-to-day consciousness. This information is usually presented to you in the form of spontaneous images and insights. You cannot make this happen; you can only establish the proper condition. The poet Rainer Maria Rilke says it this way: "Listen to the voice of the wind and the ceaseless message that forms itself in silence."

Silence is like a waterfall that connects the river above with the pool of water below. It links our day-to-day consciousness with the part of our mind that contains what is usually unavailable information, the unconscious. The moment you try to direct or analyze the information you receive, you break the silence and the linkage. In this first approach we use this capacity of the mind by first inducing silence and then quietly, nonanalytically, observing the movement of the images and insights it may generate. I say *may* because sometimes no information is forthcoming. The more skilled you become in being an observer of silence, the more success you will have.

The second approach relies on the silent mind's capacity to respond to requests for specific information, information that can provide us with insight into the issues and conflicts we would like to explore and understand more fully. This method builds on the first approach by adding direction to what previously was an undirected process. If not done carefully, presence of an objective can have a negative impact on the process. The intention must be internally stated, and then left alone in the silence. Now and then you may restate this direction, but you must immediately return to being a neutral, undemanding observer. Read through the following exercise, and then try it at an appropriate time.

1. Begin by using a method that assists you in establishing a silent mind (you can use "Accessing Inner Silence" later in this chapter). I often find that when I remain quiet for several days, in my home or elsewhere, my mind slowly quiets, providing the natural conditions for self-inquiry.

2. *When the mind is steady in silence*, become aware of any insights or new information that spontaneously arise. You may be surprised to find an unexpected insight into an issue or problem you've been concerned with. Do not seek it out. Note any thoughts or insights, but do not analyze or further process them. Just observe, in a disinterested way, the quality and extent of the images and insights that are spontaneously presented to you.

3. Next choose a concern, or idea, that you wish to explore. For example, there are times when I am writing and I seem unable to catch the essence of an idea and express it with brevity and clarity. I might present it to my silent mind in the following way: "What are the essential skills of self-exploration? I need to know them concisely, in one or two words." Your concern must be clear and circumscribed. Tell your quiet mind that you intend to receive insight into this issue. Remember, an intention is not a demand. Focus on observing your mind, not on analyzing the content. You can make a mental note and examine the information more thoroughly at another time. This is a subtle part of the process. It is as if you were watching in slow motion a flower bud unfold into a full bloom, slowly revealing its nature. As you focus your attention, continue to observe rather than dissect, analyze, or in any other way apply your intellect to this process. If you discover yourself doing this, stop, regain your silence, and begin again. Simply "plant" your objective, observe it, and allow your mind to work for you. Any insights will emerge on their own.

4. Sustain your focus and attention while maintaining a silent mind for another fifteen minutes. Again, *do not* actively analyze, explore, or mentally investigate your focal point. Just observe it with both intention and indifference while remaining silent. Observe how your mind links conscious and unconscious information. If your mind becomes active again, observe it, and when it quiets, return to your focus.

5. When and if insights come to you, note them, and do nothing more. Be patient. If this is not your time to receive further information, you can repeat the approach at another time.

6. You should continue this process for at least forty-five minutes. When forty-five minutes have elapsed, you can leave your focal point, and slowly return to the time and space of your surroundings.

Although each of us, at one time or another, has experienced spontaneous insights and understanding, it requires a considerable amount of patience and practice to develop this skill so that you can use it effectively at will. Most essential is the capacity to hold your mind in silence, and to be aware of your concern, not seeking to resolve it, but providing a space in which it can reveal itself as you look at it directly. What we are learning is quite simple: how to listen, not to our inner mental dialogue, but rather to the nonverbal essence of our being where information usually masked by our internal conversations is made available to us. What we most often receive is not detailed information, but overall understandings about ourselves, our concerns, and our direction. Developing capacities of the mind such as this often seems like staring at an optical illusion; at first, you can't see it, and then, almost suddenly, it reveals itself.

Here is an alternative approach to exploring a conscious intention in silence that uses mental imagery:

1. Begin by using a method that assists you in establishing a silent mind (again, you can use the exercise "Accessing Inner Silence" later in this chapter).

2. Next, create a visual image of an "inner adviser." This may be a person you know, a religious figure, a wise man or woman, or any other image that can serve as a counselor or adviser. When you develop this image, sit quietly in communion with it.

3. In a direct, clear, and concise manner, ask this person if you may seek assistance. If the answer is no, this is not the time, so quietly return to the time and place of your surroundings. If the answer is yes, proceed.

4. Ask your question in a direct and clear manner. Then sit in silence, neither seeking nor striving, awaiting your answer, which may come in the form of spontaneous images or in-

sights. Do not be demanding or insistent. Be patient. If the answer is to come, it will. If it doesn't, return to your adviser at another time. You may ask as many questions as your adviser is comfortable with.

5. When you have finished, acknowledge your adviser's assistance, and return to the time and place of your surroundings.

With practice you can repeat a variation of these techniques throughout the day. Place your intention in your mind and go about your other activities, now and then reminding yourself of the understandings you seek. If your mind is relatively quiet, you may find that you receive a sudden "flash" of insight.

Perhaps you have experienced this phenomenon even without the silence. Often we have a concern that won't leave our minds. We turn it over and over, examining and reexamining it to no avail, then suddenly, when we *forget* to think about it, an insight breaks through that provides all or part of the answer we need. In actuality, the mind spontaneously enters a moment of silence and then the "aha" is there.

Silence, self-inquiry, and insight help us in achieving a complete understanding of a situation rather than a partial, incomplete understanding. The knowledge that unfolds is integrative rather than analytic, and intuitive rather than intellectual. Slowly, what at first appear to be isolated discoveries congeal into larger and more systematic understandings. When we finally see into and comprehensively understand an issue or situation, we are unburdened of the tensions and conflicts associated with insufficient and limited knowledge. We "know that we know," but often don't quite know why we are so certain and clear. If we look carefully, we will notice that such breakthroughs in understanding always occur in a brief moment when the mind is still and unoccupied by the incessant inner dialogue. By cultivating the capacity for inner silence we are creating the conditions under which the truths of our lives and of nature will be revealed to us, truths that are unattainable through intellectual effort alone. This results in an inner healing, a healing at the source of both our emotional lives and our physiology.

In addition to providing understandings and guidance, these practices can be used on a regular basis to explore the sources of emotional distress. When you experience distress, don't push it away; instead allow it to dwell in your mind and body without discharging or suppressing it. Begin to observe and learn from it rather than merely reacting to it. If initially it is difficult to avoid reacting, try the following approach. The emphasis here is on first changing the intense emotion or feeling into an image, or to identify where you feel it in your body. It is important to shift your focus either to the image you have created, or to the body part where the feeling is expressed. This technique will give you some distance from the intensity of the feeling, allowing you to proceed with the exercise. The second important aspect of the exercise relies on the mind's capacity to link an emotion with your past experiences, permitting you to develop the history of this feeling—to understand the connections your mind automatically makes based on past experience. Close your eyes, sit quietly, and ask the following questions in sequence, allowing time for each of the answers.

1. *Where do I experience this distressful feeling in my body? How does it feel in this location? Does it move from place to place? Or what image comes to mind that represents this feeling? What color or shape does this feeling have?* Whether image or body feeling is stronger, focus on it, and let it unfold as you observe or experience it. If you remain a neutral observer the unconscious mind will take over and work with either the image or body feeling. Allow as much time as necessary for this to develop.

2. Next allow this image or body feeling to go back through time and develop a "history" of its presence in your life. Pro-

vide as much time as necessary. Do not "think" yourself back in time; quietly allow the feeling to find and attach itself to old circumstances.

3. Observe without judgment or interpretation any spontaneous information that may arise. [*If you are drawn back* to the intensity of the feeling, re-create an image or a body feeling and return to observing it.] When the information has ceased to flow, quietly open your eyes and reflect on your experience.

The purpose of this approach is first to gain some distance from the feeling by imagining it in the form of an image or color, and second, to use the feeling to take you toward a larger understanding of its source and significance. As you continue this exercise, your mind and body will soon quiet. Eventually, if you are patient, you will "get it"—you will see the pattern that underlies your feelings and emotions, its source, and its resolution. When this occurs, the distress is replaced by a larger understanding of yourself, the resolution of inner conflict, the reduction of stress, and the reharmonizing of your physiology. In this way the self-knowledge gained from self-exploration heals the mind and body.

What we are trying to accomplish through these practices is the development of faith and confidence in our capacity to generate from within ourselves a different kind of knowledge, knowledge about who we are, what we need, and the intention and direction that is naturally ours. Every wise man has sought his knowledge from the exact same source that is available to us: the mind and consciousness. If we, too, can learn to listen, we will hear much the same.

The exercises I have suggested are not the only ones that help us use our built-in capacities for self-inquiry and self-exploration. Reading, workshops, seminars, and psychotherapy are a few of the many other approaches. One or more may be appropriate at different moments in our lives. It is helpful to use as many resources as possible as we continuously seek to explore and understand our experiences through the changing seasons of our lives.

Once one begins to open the door to an expanded self-knowledge, the door rarely closes. When we learn to listen and observe carefully, we will be able to locate the common threads that weave through our lives. From this knowledge we will progressively align ourselves with our natural tendencies and find less and less inner and outer conflict, conflict between the inner yearnings of our natures, souls, and spirits, and the outer direction of our lives. From these insights flows healing.

When we choose to activate the Mind/Body Healing System, we shift away from a complete reliance on the automatic activity of the homeostatic system and the culturally organized practices of the treatment system. With the approaches and practices of mind/body healing we begin to take charge of our health by using our inner resources of self-regulation and by beginning the process of self-exploration, a process that will lead to an expansion of consciousness, self-knowledge, and inner harmony. Together, these two aspects of mind/body healing will provide us with the skills, confidence, and competence to reestablish our central role in self-healing.

∽

INNER JOURNEY #5: ACCESSING INNER SILENCE

This exercise will assist you in using meditation to quiet the mind. As we will explore in the next chapter, there are other ways to enter silence. However, accessing silence through meditation is a traditional and important skill to learn. It is always available, and can serve as a regular practice, assisting you in learning the skills of observation and inquiry. Begin by finding a quiet, uninterrupted space, sitting comfortably, and closing your eyes.

For the first two minutes observe your mind to determine how much and what kind of mental activity is going on. Is your inner dialogue active, or inactive? Is it worrying, planning, evaluating, or shifting from one thought, feeling, or visual image to another? *(Allow two minutes.)*

Having made this determination, begin a more careful observation of your reactive mind, the inner dialogue. As you focus, become aware of the difference between observing your mind and being possessed by it. When possessed by your active mind, you are joining with the thoughts and feelings, engaging in an active dialogue with them. You will find yourself analyzing, evaluating, interpreting, and reacting to them. We are all experts at this. It requires no further practice.

Observing the mind is quite different. It is "standing outside" of its automatic activity, thoughts, feelings, and visual images, and viewing them as if you were a disinterested spectator. This is not unlike the image of a mountain "observing" the clouds going by, or, in human terms, a reporter dispassionately observing the facts of an event. This is asking a part of you to step back, to notice without interest. This is not easy. Observe your mind in this manner for ten minutes.

If you were able to observe your mind with indifference, you will notice that however active it was when you started, it soon slowed down. It can be no other way. That is how it works. If your mind became more active, you will have learned about the tenacity of your reactive mind, which draws you to it with comments like "This is frustrating," "I can't do this," or "I'm failing again." When these thoughts arise, observe them, don't react to them. If you have difficulty, encourage your mind to be as active as it wants, while you continue to observe it. *Do not attempt to slow it down or stop it.* This will only encourage it to become more active.

If you need further assistance, create the visual image of a transparent wall separating your observing self from the active mind. You can go farther and imagine your observing self as being "miles away" from the active mind. By encouraging the active mind to "talk," separating yourself from it, restraining yourself from attempting to control it, and practicing indifferent observation, you will eventually "get it," and your mind will move toward silence.

When you have achieved inner silence, shift your observation to the movements of your chest wall and abdomen. You will notice they rise with each normal inspiration, and fall with each expiration. Begin to observe this movement. Hold your focus with sufficient intention so you don't easily wander, and at the same time not so tightly that you become tense. If your mind again becomes active with thoughts, feelings, and visual images, return to observing it as before. Remember, this training is not about the amount of silence you can create, but rather about learning the skills of observation and inquiry. Continue observing your breathing, and, when it distracts you, observe your active mind. *(Allow five minutes.)*

Next, focusing on your counting, begin counting your breath. Count 1 to 4 on the in-breath and 1 to 8 on the out-breath. Notice that the mind is naturally quieter on the out-breath. (The Yogis suggest that you experience the quietness on the out-breath and remember it on the in-breath.) Continue your counting for five minutes. Next, add a rest after the expiration. Your rhythm will now be 1 to 4 in, 1 to 8 out, and 1 to 4 rest (no breathing). Notice how your mind has little choice but to be silent when breathing stops. *(Allow five minutes.)*

Next stop breath-counting and return your focus to the rising and falling of your chest wall with inspiration and expiration. Allow your breath to diminish in frequency and volume. You are seeking to almost, comfortably, watch your breath disappear. Your breathing may become like a whisper. Notice how the mind enhances its stillness as the breath quiets. *(Allow ten minutes.)*

Next, allow your attention, while maintaining mindfulness, to shift to your body and your environment. We call this *choiceless awareness*, the capacity to be aware of all that is occurring without preference as to which you attend to and which you do not. Simply allow your mind to observe all that is happening without engaging or attaching to any one particular thing. *(Allow five minutes.)*

Become aware now of how your physiology has responded to the quieting of your mind. Your extremities may be warm and heavy (an indication of a relaxed circulatory system and increased blood flow to your skin, and relaxed musculature). Your breathing is likely softer, smoother, and diminished in intensity. Notice any other physiological changes that confirm for you the relationship of mind to body. In this manner, you can observe how the mind/body interaction goes in two directions: The mind can slow the body and the body can slow the mind.

It is now time to slowly bring your awareness back to your surroundings, opening your eyes when you are comfortable, and observing the state of your mind/body.

∾

In this exercise we have used various approaches to quieting the mind. These include using the active mind as a focal point, observing the rising and falling of the abdomen and chest with the natural breathing cycle, counting your breaths, slowing your breathing, the use of imagery, and the process of choiceless awareness. As you work with these techniques you can choose what is most helpful for you and design your meditation so that it is most comfortable, meaningful, and effective for you.

꩜

INNER JOURNEY #6:
LEARNING OBSERVATION THROUGH DAILY LIVING

I have borrowed this exercise from my earlier book, *Intentional Healing*, because I believe it offers a good example of how you can practice the skills of observation and inquiry with an activity as routine as eating. (This is a modified version of an exercise presented at a workshop by Ram Dass.) Read this exercise prior to eating a meal. Record the exercise on an audiotape, allowing thirty minutes. At the conclusion of the tape you will have an additional thirty or more minutes to complete your meal.

Place the prepared food and all that is necessary for your meal in front of you. Remain quiet in your chair for five minutes. Allow your mind and body to become still, leave the matters of the day, and focus your awareness on the eating process. The meal is to be eaten in silence over a period of one hour with slow and deliberate movements.

Begin by observing the food in front of you. Notice its shape, texture, color, and aroma. Notice how the utensils and foods play against each other. Notice the warmth or coolness of the food. Slowly choose how you will begin the meal and raise the utensil.

Place the food in your mouth and notice its texture against your body, its temperature, and its touch. Slowly chew your food, drawing your attention to all the sensations. Take as long as possible to chew the food as you experience the mechanical aspects of digestion: the movement of the jaw, teeth, and tongue; the salivary juices; the slow breakdown of the food; and the change in texture and taste. When ready, swallow the food, observing its movement into your esophagus and stomach. Pause to allow the food to digest. *(Allow five minutes.)*

You are now ready for your next mouthful of food. As you chew this mouthful, become aware of the deeper essence of the food. It incorporates the elements of the earth, the nurturing work of the farmer, and the preparation in your home, all so that you can be nourished. It is life giving to life. *(Allow five minutes.)*

You are now ready for your third mouthful. Become aware of how eating is the symbol of sacrifice. The sky sacrificed rain for the food to grow, the earth sacrificed its nutrients, the plant, its fruit. In turn we sacrifice as we serve life. *(Allow five minutes.)*

> Food is the life of all beings; and all food comes from the rain above. Sacrifice *(giving)* brings the rain from heaven, and sacrifice is sacred action.
> Sacred action ... comes from the Eternal, and therefore is the Eternal ever present in a sacrifice.
>
> —*Bhagavad Gita*

Take your next mouthful of food. Become aware of how this food, a product of the sky and the earth, will become part of the chemicals and structural elements of your mind and body. This food represents your union with all that is, and all that will be. *(Allow five minutes.)* Notice how filled you can become without a large quantity of food.

With your next mouthful experience the grace of life giving to life.

> We don't say grace *before* meals. We say it *with* meals. Or rather we don't *say* grace; we *chew it.*
> Grace is the first mouthful of each course—chewed and chewed until there is nothing left of it. And all the time you're chewing you pay attention to the flavor of the food, to its consistency and temperature, to the pressures on your teeth and the feel of the muscles in your jaws.
> [Grace is] attention to the experience of some-

thing given, something you haven't invented, not the memory of a form of words addressed to someone in your imagination.

—Aldous Huxley, *Island*

Return to the meal and continue as you have begun. Slowly, with reverence, complete your ingestion of the food *(using a total of one hour from the beginning of this exercise)*, at all times being mindful of the experience. When you have finished remain in silence for an additional five minutes, aware at all times of the present moment.

∽

As you can see from this exercise, each moment in life is an opportunity to develop mindfulness. Merely stop, become aware of the mechanical nature of your thoughts, feelings, and activities, and begin to observe them. You will always notice that when you are observing, in contrast to reacting automatically, the mind will slow and quiet as your consciousness shifts.

∽

INNER JOURNEY #7: ASSESSING SOCIAL SUPPORT

Although it is quite clear that our social interactions both enhance our capacity to resist stress and disease and encourage and directly assist us in promoting our health, it is unusual for us either to consider these experiences as activities of health, or, even less so, to measure them. This exercise will provide you the opportunity to assess carefully the quality and character of your social support system, and enable you to decide where and how it needs expansion and strengthening.

MY SOCIAL SUPPORT NETWORK

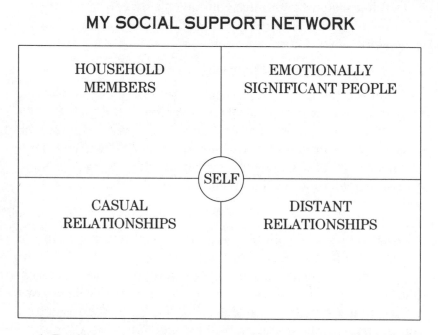

1. Begin by copying the chart above on a larger piece of paper, one that allows more space to work with.

2. Using a separate piece of paper, create four columns using each of the categories listed above as headings for the columns.

3. Under each category identify the individuals in your support system who fit into these categories, giving each a specific number (all the individuals listed should have separate numbers), and placing a circle around the females and a square around the males.

4. When the above is completed, transfer these numbers, with the circles and squares, onto their appropriate locations on the chart.

5. For a moment, observe the distribution and character of your social support system.

6. Now evaluate your network from the following perspectives:

Stability: How stable is your network? How many individuals move in and out over time? How does this affect you?

Reciprocity: Is there an equal flow of support between you and other members of your support system? In which instances does it go in one direction, or the other? Does this seem balanced and appropriate for you?

Contact Frequency: What is the frequency of contacts between you and the members of your support system? Is it sufficient or insufficient? Who initiates the contacts? Is it reciprocal?

Type of Contact: Are the contacts in person, by telephone, or by written communication? Are the contacts primarily one of information sharing, tangible assistance, or emotional sharing?

Accessibility: Are your social supports available when you need them, and in the manner you need them?

~

You may discover other ways to evaluate your social support system, and, as our social networks change, it may be valuable for you to repeat this exercise, and save and compare the results over time. Because social support is essential to healing and health, it is important that we use information such as this to evaluate the current status of our support system, and to plan to expand it in a manner that is appropriate to our needs. An active effort in this area is a critical component of Whole Healing.

THE SPIRITUAL HEALING SYSTEM

He who has a why to live for can bear with almost any how.
—Friedrich Nietzsche

Humans need meaning. It is important for us to know that life is coherent, significant, and makes sense. We also need relatedness as an antidote to the isolation and alienation of human life. The uniquely human Spiritual Healing System contributes to Whole Healing by responding to these needs in two specific ways: First, when activated through an expanded consciousness, it *enables us to discover meaning in our lives* and second, it *allows us to experience wholeness and relatedness*. Meaning and relatedness provide a path through life's adversities, guide us toward a productive and healthy life, and heal the soul and spirit.

To many people, spiritual healing does not appear to be a requirement of life; it is considered the most optional of the four healing systems, a last resort. As a result, its development requires considerable determination and effort if it is to become an effective tool for healing. There are many individuals who do not develop this healing possibility, and as a result live lives that lack the cohesiveness of meaning. Even fewer individuals use the opportunity to transcend their day-to-day lives and experience the greater unity of life. From the perspective of a practicing physician, there is little doubt that many of the mental and physical ailments of our time can be traced to an undeveloped Spiritual Healing System. Speaking of his patients over thirty-five-years old, Jung once said, "There has not been one whose problem was not that of finding a religious outlook on life. It was safe to say that every one of them felt ill because he had lost that which the living religions of every age have given to their followers, and none of them has been really healed who did not regain his religious outlook."

MEANINGFULNESS

Sandra and her family were patients in my medical practice for many years. I looked forward to Sandra's visits, her outgoing nature, wit, and sense of humor. I clearly remember the day she came to the office in her usual good mood complaining of dizzy spells. I examined her and decided to observe the symptoms over the next few days. Rather than improving, they became worse. I referred her to a neurologist. Several days later, I met Sandra and her husband in the hallway of my office building as they were leaving the neurologist's office. "What was his opinion?" I asked. With a strange casualness that sometimes accompanies a sudden shock, she responded, "The tests show that I have brain cancer, and I will have to be operated on next week." The operation took place, and was followed by chemotherapy and radiation therapy, all to no avail. Within weeks her condition rapidly declined. First there was the loss of eyesight in one eye, then a paralysis below the waist, weight loss, profound fatigue, and endless pain. Sandra spent the last two months of her life in a nursing facility.

As I relate this story I can feel the sadness of her death return to me, a sadness that I never witnessed in Sandra. "I have had a good life," she would say, "and if it is my time to explore the other side then I'm ready to go. I would just like to stay around until my husband and children have enough time to accommodate to my death, and then I will leave. There are plans for me that I don't yet understand." Everyone who visited her went in with sadness, but left at peace. Toward the end of Sandra's life I saw her husband in my office. He finally seemed accepting of his wife's death, had gained some weight, and was sleeping better. Two days after this visit, with her family present, Sandra died peacefully. She had found meaning in her life, and meaning in her death. Though she was not cured in the conventional sense, she had been healed.

Finding meaning in the adversities and transitions of our lives requires a considerable amount of consciousness. In our discussions of the individual healing systems we have already seen how an expanding consciousness allows us to apply more and more of our inner capacities toward healing. But as our consciousness develops, it increasingly begins to ask different questions about life, questions such as, Who am I? Where am I going? What is my life about? What is the meaning of life? At one time or another it is almost certain that each of us will struggle with these concerns.

Ironically, it is only through an even further expansion of consciousness that we can find the answers to these questions, answers that can heal the disquiet these questions bring to our lives. Intuitive consciousness, a characteristic of the Spiritual Healing System, helps us to penetrate and reach beyond the details of our day-to-day experiences to apprehend patterns, relationships, and wholeness that bring meaning to life.

As humans we face the dilemma of finding meaning in a world that no longer conveys it to us. Primitive man felt a sense of connectedness with life. For him, meaning emerged from his day-to-day contact and struggle with nature. In the modern era, there were times when religious systems accomplished this task for us. But now the scientific worldview, with its microscopes and telescopes that can penetrate all matter, has stripped meaning from the universe. These instruments have left us with a devitalized world. To a large extent Nietzsche was correct in his famous statement, "The gods are dead." It is now quite difficult to discover meaning outside of ourselves. In Joseph Campbell's words, "Today no meaning is in the group—none in the world: all is in the individual."

In a very practical sense this is the normal daily fare in an internist's office. Whatever the ailment, whether it be anxiety or heart disease, one often finds it is accompanied by a sense of meaninglessness: marriage without love, work without passion, the emptiness of daily routines, the powerlessness of modern living, and the alienation and isolation of urban living. Most of us have little time for our families, less time for our friends, and no time for ourselves. We move from task to task in a seemingly disconnected way with few if any interludes for contemplating our situation. These are the circumstances that underlie illness, and rob us of a healthy life. They are not the concern of the Homeostatic Healing System, where meaninglessness does not threaten our internal balance in the usual sense, nor of a treatment system that cannot treat what it cannot feel or touch, nor even of the Mind/Body Healing System, whose efforts are directed toward the mechanics of self-regulation and the dynamics of psychological development. So where do we begin?

Although there are many places we can look for meaning, among which are service to others, commitment to loved ones, dedication to a cause, creativity, self-actualization, and transcendent beliefs, we cannot find meaning merely by looking. It doesn't come that way. We can only find it by engaging life as it presents itself to us in the present moment. What does this mean? It means that *wherever I am, whatever I am doing, that is where I need to find meaning.* I must look below the surface of my experiences and intuit how they relate to and are linked to my life. There is perhaps no better example of how this is done than in the life of the psychiatrist Viktor Frankl. A prisoner in Auschwitz from 1943 to 1945, he was a witness to unbearable pain and suffering. His personal response bears repeating here:

> When a man finds that it is his destiny to suffer, he will
> have to accept his suffering as his task: his single and
> unique task. He will have to acknowledge the fact that
> even in suffering he is unique and alone in the universe.
> No one can relieve him from his suffering or suffer in his
> place. His unique opportunity lies in the way in which he
> bears his burden.

Frankl related his experiences in his book *Man's Search for Meaning*, and developed a form of psychotherapy called logotherapy, which seeks to help the individual discover meaning in his or her life. He taught us that we often cannot choose what life gives us, but we can always choose how to respond to it—we can always discover meaning within our circumstances, however dark they may seem. Again, in Frankl's words:

> The last of the human freedoms is to choose one's attitude in a given set of circumstances, to choose one's way.
> It is this spiritual freedom that cannot be taken away that
> makes life meaningful and purposeful.

As a physician, I most often meet patients in the context of disease. So disease is where we begin. As we have followed Marie throughout our discussion of the healing systems, I would like to use her as an example again. As you may recall from our first discussion, I asked Marie a simple question: "What happened to the guilt, anger, and sadness related to your mother's death?" It was a question she couldn't answer, and would not be able to answer until she could begin to view her disease less as an external imposition by allergens, and more as a vital part of her life. In our search to find meaning in her current circumstance, there are other questions that I will, at the right time, raise with her. I would like to ask them now in a more general way so that they can be helpful to the reader.

Let's begin with some open-ended questions, questions that are concerned with the issue of meaning and purpose. Rather than reading through these questions one time quickly, try to spend a day reflecting and meditating on each of them, and then write your thoughts, of whatever length, in a journal.

My work is _____
My family is _____
My relationships are _____
Each day is _____
Life to me seems _____
If I had my choice I would _____
For me, life means _____
If I died today my life would have been _____

Do the answers to these questions leave you satisfied that your life has meaning and direction, or not? Please remember that meaning can be found even at times of chaos and despair if you can simply see a reason, a purpose in it—something you can make of it. So if you discover from these questions that your life seems unsatisfying, accept that as what is happening to you at this moment. Find meaning in that dissatisfaction. Is it to motivate you to further action? Is it to awaken your spirit and soul? Is it to inform you about your true nature, and any changes you must make in your life's circumstances? What can you learn from this stage of your life—patience, persistence, or another trait?

I would next focus more specifically on the symptoms and characteristics of disease. Variations of these same questions can be applied to whatever circumstance concerns you at the present moment. Again, consider the questions carefully and write your thoughts down. Use your imagination to structure these questions to fit your situation.

Why did this disease-disorder-distress begin when it did?
How does it relate to my life?
What does it tell me about my life?
Is there any good that will come from it?
How can I find meaning in what appears meaningless?
How has it shown me the ways my life must change?

Over the period of my relationship with patients some of these questions and others would naturally arise during our conversations. They may be explored in dialogue, through recommended readings, meditation, imagery, art, dance, drama, and many other potential forums. Our exploration will be a beginning with no real end. The patient's disease is our starting point; his or her life is the core of the issue. Each individual, with his or her concern, style, and temperament, guides the dialogue, defines the questions, and brings a uniqueness to the exploration of meaning. This is a long-term, dynamic process. Life changes with time, and old meanings must give way to newer ones. The entire process is an intuitive one, which at times may overlap with the self-exploration aspect of the Mind/Body Healing System. When dealing with real-life issues, the distinctions between the systems begin to dissolve.

Whatever your concern is, begin there, and after you are finished cursing the gods, ask the critical question. It is never an accident that we find ourselves in the circumstances that we do, *and it may not be a direct result of attitudes or actions on your part.* Adversity is there to help shape us, define us, grow our character, and above all inform us. Whether we are dealing with a disease, a difficult relationship, stress at work, or unbearable financial problems, as individuals we must bring meaning to bear on our afflictions.

The Spiritual Healing System allows us to penetrate the immediacy of our problems and to intuit the patterns and relationships that convey meaning. And we are discovering, through the empirical work of Frankl and others, the clinical investigations of researchers such as Antonovsky and Kobassa, and those who are defining the mechanics that connect mind, body, and spirit, that meaning and health are closely intertwined.

WHOLENESS

Not long ago, on a small East Coast barrier island, I had the opportunity to watch with my daughters, Ali and Jessie, the great sea turtles as they reenacted their age-old ritual of leaving the sea, depositing their eggs in the sand, and retracing their steps back to their natural home. Meticulously, they followed an unchanging process that requires the digging of a nest, release of the eggs, covering of the nest, and a return to the sea. Although the sea turtles' entire lives are otherwise spent in the water, for millions of years they have carried out, with little deviation, this wondrous ritual of nature.

For me this was a spiritual experience, an experience of wholeness. I know it because I felt it. However, communicating it through words is a far more difficult task. If I am speaking to you about my body, you will know exactly what I am speaking about because the body can be directly experienced through the senses; it can be seen and touched. When we speak about feelings, attitudes, and perceptions, the elements of psychology, communication begins to get more difficult. These mental experiences cannot be known directly through the senses. Yet, we can "see" them indirectly through our behavior, and through the eyes of others who can provide us with feedback about ourselves. But when we begin to speak about spirituality we are in a far more subtle area, one that is inaccessible to the senses and largely inaccessible to words. If there is a best way to communicate this experience it is through the eyes of the artist, poet, and musician. However, art does not actually communicate this experience; rather, it evokes it within us.

Evoking a sense of the spiritual through words is a far more difficult effort, and, to some extent, communicating in such a way relies upon my readers already having had a sense of what such an experience is like. Fortunately, at one time or another we have all had a glimpse of wholeness. Much as the body develops with an inborn knowledge of its basic mechanisms, the mind also develops with built-in information. From birth, it contains a knowledge of wholeness. We each carry this knowledge in the recesses of our minds. When this remembrance is evoked within us we reexperience it, for a few moments or a few hours. Meditation, prayer, art, nature, love, music, and the aesthetic can each evoke this sense. This human capacity is universal. As a result, all cultures have expressed the spiritual experience in one form or another.

In history and literature wholeness has been called by many names. In the alchemical tradition it has been called the *coniunctionis*, the conjunction of mind, body, and spirit. In the ancient Greek tradition it is called the sacred marriage and the hierosgamos, the union of psychological opposites, for example, male and female. It is symbolized by the grail, the cup of the Last Supper, which holds abundance; the mandala, the universal image that relates the outer circumference of a circle to its inner center; and the lapis philosophorum, the alchemical factor that catalyzes the union of opposites. In the religious tradition it is symbolized by the Star of David and the Christian cross. The Western psychologist Abraham Maslow calls it self-actualization, the end point of self-development; the alchemists call it the gold, the wholeness achieved at the end of their work; Buddhism calls it the no-self, the self that has no name, characteristics, or qualities; Christianity calls it grace, and Yoga calls it enlightenment. Whatever the symbol or name, it is the same. The very fact that the knowledge of wholeness has been described with remarkable similarity in diverse cultures throughout the ages provides us with a certainty that wholeness is an enduring aspect of the human experience.

The experience of wholeness has several characteristics: It

is never about day-to-day details or events, it is always a highly
personal experience, and it is at all times accompanied by a
profound feeling of certainty, absolute truth, peacefulness, ex-
pansiveness, and timelessness. It can only be experienced in
the silence between thoughts. Wholeness can be experienced
as a sudden flash of insight, or one that is intentionally developed. It is not meant as a final resting place, but rather as a
touchstone of what is possible. In this way it offers a certain
perspective to our day-to-day lives, what we would call a transcendent perspective—a broad overview. This perspective
provides a larger context for our lives, one that can help us
link together our many experiences, our joys, losses, and transitions, into one understandable whole. And this whole, we
discover, is part of a larger whole. Einstein expressed this in
the following way:

> A human being
> is a part of the whole,
> called by us,
> "Universe": a part limited
> in time and space.
> He experiences himself,
> his thoughts and feelings,
> as something separated
> from the rest—
> a kind of optical delusion
> of his consciousness.
> This delusion
> is a kind of prison for us,
> restricting us
> to our personal desires
> and to affection
> for a few persons nearest us.
> Our task must be
> to free ourselves
> from this prison.

As a physician regularly consulting with patients I routinely ask myself when and how to make use of this healing system, how to assist individuals with both discovering meaning in their lives and experiencing wholeness and its transcendent perspective. It took me many years to develop a respect for the human life cycle, to know that there are tasks for each part of life and specific resources we must bring to bear on these tasks. I have found that the capacity to bring a spiritual perspective into one's life is linked to two variables: age and receptiveness. The tasks in the early part of life are largely that of formal education, socialization, career, and family. These are very human day-to-day endeavors that generally proceed at their own pace without a perceived need for a spiritual perspective. It is toward the middle of life and beyond, when we most confront disease, aging, and mortality, that spirituality becomes less of a luxury. The major issues of this part of life rarely resolve themselves without a sustained use of the four healing systems available to us. Regardless of age, some individuals are receptive to the resources of this healing system and some are not. Adversity, a certain maturity, and an inquisitive and open mind enhance an individual's interest in the spiritual perspective.

The use of certain techniques or conditions can potentially evoke the momentary experience of wholeness. In fact, this is rather easy to accomplish. But only through the long-term commitment to self-development and to the expansion of consciousness can we meaningfully use the Spiritual Healing System. Many of the activities previously mentioned—meditation, silence, nature, music and art, among others—can assist in evoking a feeling of wholeness. But it has been my experience that these approaches, unlinked to self-development and the expansion of consciousness, rarely have lasting impact, and therefore, although they may serve as a touchstone for future growth and development, they do not serve to activate the Spiritual Healing System.

Wholeness is progressively arrived at in a manner that can

best be termed *integration and reconciliation*. The goal of self-knowledge, the aim of the Mind/Body Healing System, is to arrive at a full understanding of ourselves. Such an understanding includes both a knowledge of the more apparent parts of our character and, of most importance, an understanding of what Jung called our "shadow" side, the fears, anxieties, and unacceptable qualities that, although absent from our day-to-day view, exert a powerful influence on our behavior and our lives.

For example, in Marie's life, feelings of guilt and anger over her mother's death are fairly well suppressed. I imagine that they have a long history dating back to childhood. To the extent that they are suppressed rather than considered and dealt with, they will express themselves in ways unrecognizable to Marie—in her case a persistent anxiety and the emergence of asthma. The process of self-exploration will "shine a flashlight" on these aspects of her character, and in this way integrate them into her life in a manner that precludes their expression in unhealthy ways. To integrate and reconcile ourselves with all of our qualities allows inner harmony to displace inner conflict. The more harmony we naturally bring to our lives, the more silent the mind and the more open we are to the experience of wholeness on a day-to-day basis. As we can see, the activation of the Spiritual Healing System is closely allied to the development of mind/body healing.

The *Eumenides,* by the ancient Greek poet/playwright Aeschylus, is a story that beautifully expresses the necessary integration and reconciliation that evokes and sustains wholeness. Orestes, chased by the Furies of Shame and Guilt, arrives in the city of Athens. As some may know, in the first two books of this trilogy Orestes conspires with his sister Electra in the revengeful murder of their mother, Clytemnestra, who herself had taken on a lover and killed her husband, King Agamemnon, the father of Orestes and Electra, upon his return from the Trojan wars. Tormented by Shame and Guilt, Orestes bids the assistance of the wise goddess Athena. Athena, in the spirit of democracy, suggests the very first jury trial. Orestes will have a chance to explain his predicament and his wish to be released from the torment of the Furies, and the Furies will similarly have their say. The trial is held and the jury finds in favor of Orestes, who, they feel, has suffered long enough. The Furies, in a fit of rage, insist that in revenge for this finding they will forever curse the city of Athens.

It is at this point that Athena teaches us the process of reconciliation, the act of integrating all of the aspects of our selves into a coherent, unified whole.

To Orestes she has given peace. To the Furies she next offers an honored home as important citizens of Athens. They will be consulted about all major decisions and will be respected and cared for by their fellow citizens. In return, they must honor, bless, and become participants in the community of Athens. After some questioning and reassurance, they accept, the integration is complete, and unity and peace return.

How important it is for us to remember that stories and myths, which have never "happened," are in fact psychological truths. Much as the wise Athena, we must learn how to negotiate between our opposing inner voices, integrating them all and respecting their important places in our lives as honored citizens in a diverse inner civilization.

There are several steps I follow when assisting an individual in moving toward a more sustained experience of oneness. I begin by teaching one or more of the quieting techniques that we have previously discussed. Most often I begin with meditation. Meditation provides the inner silence and context through which an individual can develop and expand self-knowledge and consciousness. From the beginning I make it very clear that the ultimate goal of this practice is neither the short-term gain of relaxation nor the interim and important expansion of self-knowledge, but rather the capacity to experience wholeness, a seamless inner and outer relatedness. As we progress, I will usually offer suggestions regarding readings, workshops, and seminars that may assist with this process. Our ongoing dialogue is a mutual one as we explore together new insights, discoveries, and the important questions and issues that arise on the way to a more informed self.

There are certain lifestyles that can assist you in activating the Spiritual Healing System as well. First, it is important to allow for a sufficient level of solitude—time alone with oneself. It is only in this way that we can have the uninterrupted opportunity to still the mind, and experience, observe, and reflect upon our lives. It is quite easy to avoid time alone, as life provides us with more than enough important obligations and trivial distractions. At times we need to retreat for several days, while at other times we may need no more than a brief break in our day-to-day activities. I have usually found that after just a few days of silence, I can begin to feel a certain inner quiet and peacefulness, which allows for a more novel and accurate look at the issues in my life.

Second, I recommend a minimum of clutter in one's life. Simplicity and austerity help to minimize the too often frenetic pace of our lives, a pace that is inconsistent with our natural rhythms and detrimental to the conditions that are necessary for the development of consciousness. The issue here is making a distinction between what we think we want and what we truly need.

Finally, peaceful relationships make for a more silent mind. I frequently recall Patanjali's advice to Yoga students in the *Yoga Sutras*: Have goodwill toward those that are healthy, compassion toward those that are ill, and benign indifference toward those that would do you harm. It was good advice then, and it's good advice now.

As we exercise spiritual healing, change can often be seen within a short period of time. First, there is less reactiveness toward others, and a calmer attitude toward daily life. With this increased quiet new insights and observations arise. Not only do we see our own behavior more clearly, but we also see that of others. We see the ways we navigate our lives: pleasing others for approval, creating distance for safety, manipulating through giving, seeking attention by playing victim, and so on. As we uncover these childhood strategies we begin to discover the fears, sadness, and hurt that underlie the development of these patterns. As we look directly at these parts of ourselves we begin to reconcile ourselves with their presence and integrate them into our inner community, and in this process they lose their potency, which, as in the case of the Furies, they give up in order to live in the light of day. Over time there is more of a sense of self inside of us. Confidence is gained, there is less concern with the approval or disapproval of others, and an expanding sense of self-reliance and inner harmony. This is not the work of a weekend or week. It is a long-term undertaking whose results become evident almost from the start.

When the work of mind/body healing is well on its way, wholeness begins to emerge from within. Through an understanding of the particulars of our lives we discover the universal patterns and truths; through an exploration of the apparent world we discover essence. As I have said, these revelations rarely happen all at once—they arrive piece-by-piece as a series of direct personal discoveries. Slowly the veil lifts, permitting us to see life as it is. We have all experienced aspects of this. It is the "aha" experience, the feeling that "I know that I know," a release of tension, a slow, yet certain emergence of a feeling of completion, a return of vitality, and an enlargement of self. Jung states it this way:

> Only one who has risked the fight with the dragon and is not overcome by it wins the hoard, the "treasure hard to attain." He alone has a genuine claim to self-confidence, for he has faced the dark ground of himself and thereby has gained himself. This experience gives him faith and trust, the *pistis* in the ability of the self to sustain him, for everything that has menaced him from inside he has made his own. He has acquired the right to believe that he will be able to overcome all future threats by the same means. He has arrived at an inner certainty that makes

him capable of self-reliance, and attained what the alchemists call the *unio mentalis.*

The development of spirituality is not meant to remove us
from our daily lives, but rather to expand them. It is easy to im-
merse ourselves exclusively in our day-to-day lives, and it is
equally possible to isolate ourselves in the spiritual experience. It is bringing them together that is difficult. We are both
spirit and soul, and wholeness resides in their union, not in
their separateness. For this to happen, spirit must join soul.
Soul is composed of the elements of our day-to-day life: our
emotions, images, dreams, pain, suffering, and joy. Soul is of
the body. It is in the rich experience of the complexity and fullness of our humanity that we experience soulfulness. Spirit is
of a different nature. It has a transcendent quality, one that
overlooks life, viewing it as a whole. Spirit is unconcerned
with details. It is concerned with the cosmic and the divine.
Where soul brings us deep into the guts of life, spirit takes us
away from these issues. Soul has been described as horizontal,
of the earth, and feminine. Spirit has been described as horizontal, of the sky, and masculine. Spirit, once developed, is
meant to spiritualize soul—our daily lives; and soul, in return,
humanizes our spirit—our link to the divine. And it is their
union that pleases the intellect, nurtures the soul, elevates the
spirit, and transforms and revitalizes our lives. In this way the
Spiritual Healing System heals at the source. Anything less is
partial healing.

Wholeness and unity as experienced by the undeveloped
infant and the maturing adult differs in only one respect.
The infant, as a result of his undifferentiated consciousness, is
a participant in a primal unity. The mature adult experiences
precisely the same unity and wholeness, with one exception,
he or she knows it. For some, this awareness may seem a
small difference for which to spend a life exploring and enduring tension and suffering. But this is our divine spark, our
uniqueness and destiny as humans, one that distinguishes us

from all other forms of life and perhaps conveys to us the responsibility to articulate, preserve, and honor nature's intentions. The entire movement toward wholeness is patterned into our minds: First we must separate from the unconscious unity of infancy, then we must develop pyschologically and expand our consciousness, and, finally, we will increasingly experience our wholeness. It is perhaps best expressed in the well-known lines from T. S. Eliot's *The Four Quartets:*

> We shall never cease exploring
> and when we will arrive at our destination
> we will have returned to the same place
> only to know it for the first time. . . .

CLOSE ONE DOOR
AND OPEN ANOTHER

When I had journeyed half of my life's way,
I found myself within a shadowed forest,
For I had lost the path that does not stray.
—Dante, *Inferno*

In the preceding chapters we set out to explore the broad out-
lines of Whole Healing. When we shift from using only one
healing system to the resources of Whole Healing, there is a
corresponding change in our ideas about health and disease.
Where previously we considered only one view of health and
disease, the view of the treatment system, we can now consider a more expansive view, the view of Whole Healing. When
it comes to health, our old beliefs, thoughts, feelings, and images will be replaced by new ones.

From this changed perspective, health is no longer viewed
as a singular experience, a static condition or state of being. It
is dynamic, vital, and multidimensional, and includes each of
the four healing systems: the maintenance of internal balance,
the repair and restoration of normal function, the expansion of
consciousness and the development of the skills and resources
of self-regulation, and the achievement of wholeness. From

this viewpoint, health is a personal endeavor that is a central and consistent part of our lives. It is not only defined by normal laboratory results and regular physical exams, but also by the way we succeed in growing throughout our lives. In sum, health is seen more as a *verb* than a *noun*, a dynamic activity and attitude rather than a fixed, definable condition. Whole Health is something we can only do for ourselves. It is not given; it is developed. It is an ongoing journey.

In our culture we are not taught to think about this journey, but rather about the limited destination of the treatment system with its exclusive focus on the notions of disease and repair. If we are to consider a revitalized vision of health we must begin by redefining and expanding our relationship with disease, bringing it into accord with the principles of Whole Healing.

Within the framework of the treatment system, we are taught that disease, when it "strikes" us, is a sort of intermission in our lives that begins with the appearance of distress and ends with its disappearance. Beyond disrupting our well-laid plans, we neither believe nor act as if this intrusion was in any way linked to either our past or our future. It is not part of the story line of our lives, but rather an unpleasant and undesirable interruption to be disposed of as rapidly as possible. This is the way we have learned to "objectify" disease, depersonalizing and defining it in a way that shapes it for the limited interventions of the treatment system. In the early years of my practice, many of the patients I saw in my office would, in a sense, bring the "disease" to me as if it were a separate entity wrapped in a box to be left with me until I treated and fixed it, somewhat like leaving one's car at the service station: "Just let me know what has to be done, and the price, and I'll pick it up when it's fixed." For us, disease has little significance or meaning beyond its intrusiveness. We merely seek to be rid of it.

We also learn to react to disease in a specific way. We respond with certain feelings and emotions, and retain certain images that are a direct consequence of the treatment system.

These must be recognized if we are to shift toward Whole Healing. In my workshops, I ask participants to join me in the following exercise in order to access this personal information. I suggest that you follow the instructions and try it for yourself.

Find a comfortable seat and close your eyes. Spend a few moments quieting your mind in whatever manner works best for you. (If you have never tried to quiet your mind before, try this by taking ten deep breaths while counting from 1 to 4 while breathing in and from 1 to 8 while breathing out.) Then try to remember your first experience of disease, either your own or that of a loved one. Take yourself back to this time as if you were actually there, and allow yourself to experience the old feelings and emotions. Explore this experience as long as it continues to provide you with new information.

Next take yourself to other encounters with disease and distress and further explore your thoughts, feelings, and images. When you've done this, explore what your images of disease would be, as if you were choosing photographs for a book on disease. Allow your images to pass before you.

When you have viewed your images, imagine that you are ready to write your book on disease. Give this book a name, think about the chapters it would include, and insert your images into your imaginary book.

When you have completed this exercise open your eyes and actually write the title, chapter ideas, and list of your photographs on a sheet of paper.

When I ask the workshop participants to share their experience the information comes quite rapidly. "I learned that disease made me feel powerlessness, helplessness, and great fear." "I felt isolated and alone." "It was one of the few times I received attention and affection." "Disease is blackness. It's filled with dread."

Examine your own experiences of disease. How were they similar and how were they different? Although the specifics may vary, it is likely that most of us will view disease as a very negative intrusion in our lives, one that is filled with fear, helplessness, and despair and whose presence is an unwanted and a purposeless distraction from our usual activities.

The treatment system similarly defines our ideas about health. We can explore these ideas through another simple exercise, which I suggest you try now.

Close your eyes and take yourself back to a moment in time when you felt completely healthy. Pay attention to the sights and sounds, and completely reexperience this time in your life. If you cannot remember such a moment, create it in your imagination as you would imagine it to be. Allow yourself five to ten minutes to experience this moment of health fully, observing its qualities and its characteristics.

In my workshops, this experience is easily and enthusiastically shared. "It was a moment of freedom and naturalness." "Everything seemed connected, vibrant, and full of delight." "I felt fully alive, alert, and peaceful." Like disease, health is often viewed as an event or condition, a particularly pleasurable moment in time that seems to arise unpredictably and leave in much the same way, a preferred state of being that moves in and out of our lives in a largely random manner. It is both the absence of disease and a positive feeling of delight and pleasure. In either case, as appealing as health is, we seem to have little understanding of or control over the factors that bring it about, or any ability to sustain it beyond its allotted time other than following some general avoidance or preventive strategies. The fact is, we are accustomed to accepting health simply as good feelings that come and go, rather than as something we can consciously sustain on our own.

These are our usual notions about health and disease. Because we are trained in this viewpoint, most of us never stray from these conventional concepts. Yet these limited views, something as intangible as an idea, can actually enhance our risk of disease and diminish our potential for health. And although it may be currently fashionable to distance ourselves from these viewpoints by pointing to our many "health"-oriented activities—our good habits, our stated beliefs in wellness and holism, and our efforts toward that end—when we look carefully at how we allocate our time and resources, we see that where health is concerned, our priorities and actions continue to be directed toward avoiding or eradicating disease, and maintaining and restoring function rather than achieving Whole Health. Despite what we say, or think we believe, when we set our priorities, make the difficult choices, and spend time and energy, we continue, in one way or another, to act out the definition of health and disease that is limited to the treatment system.

Consider how most of us would answer the simple question I put to patients looking for a new road to health: "Can you set aside just one hour a day for meditation or exercise?" The most frequent response is "Where am I going to find the time?" Next I ask, "If I told you right now that you were ill and needed to be in the hospital for three weeks would you find the time?" The answer is always, "Of course." Finally, when I ask whether it would be possible to take three weeks off to focus completely on health, the answer comes only after a long pause: "Well . . . maybe . . . Not now . . . I need to think about it. . . ." and so on. What would your answer be? The reality is that most of us must still get ill before we are motivated to get well, and we rarely allocate time or financial resources to health activities as readily as we do to the care of disease. Many people would argue that it would be difficult to take time off from work unless something is noticeably "wrong." It is undeniable that our culture legitimizes and makes it easier to pursue disease-related activities rather than Whole Health.

A NEW VISION OF DISEASE AND HEALTH

What we have learned about health and disease is limited and does not serve us well—in fact, in the long run it may make us sick. Let's reconsider the issue of disease. To see disease as we are compelled to by our inherited worldview is to misdiagnose its role in our life. According to our new view, disease is a personal experience, an amalgam of objective change and subjective experiences. However unwanted it may be, it is part of our lives that brings meaning and purpose with it. When it is present in our lives it can be a master teacher that can inform us about life and initiate the process of Whole Healing. It is a break with the ordinary, a crack in the egg (or should I say on the head!) that tells us all is not right.

Despite what we have been taught, *disease and distress can point the way and serve as a transition to an expanded and revitalized life.* By activating the Mind/Body and Spiritual Healing Systems it can be one of the most instructive periods in our lives. It can be an open doorway, an important opportunity, not one that we seek, but one that nevertheless may be given to us. When this opportunity is missed, it may not reappear for decades. Life will go on, but it will do so in a contracted and limited manner. Not to move through this open doorway is a tragic loss. Perhaps there can be no greater condemnation of the treatment system than its consistent habit of closing the doorway to this opportunity for growth, development, meaning, and change by treating disease exclusively with surgery, pharmaceuticals, and practices, without recognizing its larger meaning, purpose, and possibilities.

Let's look at our ideas about disease from the perspective of the health continuum. As we move through the initial loss and suffering of disease we have a choice. We can automatically return to our learned reactions to illness, powerlessness, helplessness, fear, and withdrawal (feelings and actions that may actually worsen the disease), or we can view disease as a dynamic aspect of our lives. In this manner we can shift our perspectives and try to understand the meaning and significance of this experience while simultaneously developing and expanding our personal skills and resources and extending our healing capacities. From this vantage point, we must be willing to see how disease fits into the story line of our lives. We must ask ourselves important questions such as:

- What are the factors in my mind-set and lifestyle that have influenced the development of this illness?

- What does it tell me about my work, relationships, level of stress, and chosen way of life? How have these factors influenced my health?

- What are the resources I can draw upon, and the new capacities and skills I will now need?

- What meaning can I discover in this illness that will give it value and significance in my life?

- What will it require for me to see this illness as a challenge rather than a source of despair?

- How will this illness help shape the next years of my life?

Beyond assisting us in understanding and reorganizing our lives, discovering the meaning of this unexpected disruption helps us to move through it—a fact we are beginning to discover in our investigations of the role of positive emotions in the mind/body connection. Further, experiencing disease as a vital part of our life process allows us to "make sense" of what would otherwise appear to be a senseless experience. We have learned from the experience of concentration-camp survivors and others who have moved through severe adversity that finding meaning and purpose in adversity enhances one's capacity to endure and survive. Perhaps this sentiment was best expressed by Nietzsche when he suggested that when there is a why, there is always a how. The decision to view disease as an integral part of our lives, an important message and statement, is an important first step in activating the Mind/Body and Spiritual Healing Systems. It begins to shift us from an exclusive dependency on treatment to an expanded set of options for both recovery and personal transformation.

Many years ago Michael came to my office with symptoms that resembled those of ulcerative colitis. After the appropriate tests were done, we were sure of the diagnosis. Although he suffered from many unpleasant and uncomfortable symptoms, he insisted that he did not want to use medications. He asked me to assist him with nonpharmacological approaches to his disease. I let him know that this would require considerable effort, and that most likely it would also require significant changes in his life. He responded, "Let's begin."

We started with meditation, a practice that became a regular part of Michael's routine. We then began to talk about the stress in his life, in his case, both work and marital stress. Within several months it became evident to him that meditation was not enough; he realized that he needed to deal directly with these sources of stress. He immediately spoke with his supervisor about his workload and need for better communication about what was expected of him. With these clarified goals, he was able to make some helpful changes at work. He next began marital therapy to resolve issues of balancing his career and family responsibilities more successfully. Eighteen months later, his marriage was remarkably improved, his work situation was stabilized, and his symptoms were gone. I haven't seen Michael for eight years, but every now and then I receive a letter from him with a list of meditation study groups and centers in our local area, a list he knows I will pass on to others. The letter always ends the same way, *Doing well, thanks!—Michael.*

Michael discovered that once he decided to see his illness as a *challenge*, he found many new resources, both inner and outer. He began to learn about his mind, and how he could use it for self-regulation, recovery, and health. With meditation, he took the first step in reconnecting mind, body, and spirit, a step that was essential for Whole Healing. Practices such as Yoga, meditation, biofeedback, breathing exercises, and body awareness, among others, may become important new resources for the recovery and the promotion of health (see "Resources" at the end of this book). As in Michael's case, disease, the thing we most dread, can serve as a powerful influence, one that can initiate a healing process that starts with the disease, yet ends with Whole Healing. In this way we view disease as an opportunity rather than as an adversity. This is not to say that we seek out disease for its opportunities, but rather that when it occurs we seek a meaning in it that enables us to use it to revitalize our lives. Disease becomes a positive agent for Whole Health, rather than a source of negative and defeating emotions and actions.

Much the same can be said of our ideas about health. We were taught that health is a condition that comes and goes rather haphazardly. This view of health, like our learned view of disease, serves us poorly. Let's look at it from a new and different perspective, one that has a very different meaning and direction. This revitalized perspective offers us the view that health is something we do for ourselves, not something that is done *to* us, a journey rather than a destination, a dynamic, holistic, and purposeful way of living.

What does this lifetime journey look like? As we see in the figure below, it is a continuous process of growth and development, which slowly leads us from a life lived on automatic pilot toward an expanding awareness, self-realization, and wholeness—the final goals of healing. The capacity to shift from the autoregulation of homeostasis, to reparative techniques, to self-regulation, and finally to a fully conscious life is built into the human mind, but we must choose to activate this shift. Thus we can choose to let circumstances carry us along, or approach health as the process that it is, thus actively developing and creating a healthy life.

WHOLENESS

Coherence

Creativity

Autonomy

Resourcefulness

Commitment

Self-knowledge

Awareness

AUTOMATICITY

Health is a process, a lifelong orientation that progressively moves us from a more or less automated existence to a life of awareness, self-knowledge, autonomy, creativity, and wholeness.

Viewing health as a process, we may ask, What are some of the specific activities that lead us along this continuum? To begin with, there is a certain kind of caring we can bring to our existence, a caring and attention that assists us in actively shaping the character of our lives. Caring mixed with curiosity propels us toward an exploration of our lives, a self-inquiry that progressively expands our consciousness and self-knowledge. This enlarging self-knowledge can further assist us in identifying the factors that lead us toward health, developing important new skills, and gathering essential resources that are necessary to activate the Mind/Body and Spiritual Healing Systems. Underlying each of these is the most essential activity we must engage in if we are to seek a life of health: the expansion of consciousness.

When we consider the larger issue of Whole Healing, we discover that health is more than extending life, preventing or curing disease, or developing the capacity for self-regulation. Although each of these goals is worthy, Whole Healing has an entirely different direction and meaning, one that incorporates but goes beyond each of these more limited goals. This is similar to recognizing that life includes our hearts pumping, our cells dividing, and our glands secreting hormones, but it is more than these physiological activities.

Health is a *way of living* that values personal growth and development, not as an antidote to disease, but for its own sake. This is a difficult concept to "catch." It requires that we suspend our usual way of thinking about the specific goals of each healing system and consider health as an active, ongoing process. We are involved in the process of health when we are proactively responding to life by adapting, growing, and expanding our awareness, resources, and capacities. The individual healing systems support this process, but they are not in themselves the whole story.

HEALTH FOR HEALTH'S SAKE

Several years ago, John, a fifty-three-year-old engineer, was referred to my office by his cardiologist. He had recently suffered a heart attack and undergone an angioplasty, a procedure that mechanically strips the cholesterol plaques obstructing blood flow in the coronary vessels. In our initial visit, we spoke for a considerable period of time, during which I informed him of the possibility that through major dietary change, exercise, the reduction of stress, and a reevaluation of his mental state and lifestyle, he could directly influence the healing of his coronary heart disease. I provided him with the appropriate information and scheduled a follow-up appointment. A week later I received a letter from him in which he explained that he was canceling his appointment, as he wished a more "conventional" approach to his disease. He had been conditioned to think that the treatment system was the only approach.

Steve, a construction contractor, arrived in my office with much the same history as John. Following our discussion, I made a similar set of recommendations. In contrast to John,

Steve actively took charge, changing his diet, exercising regularly, and directly confronting the conflicts and stress in his life. He started attending a Yoga class, entered counseling with his wife, and began to practice relaxation techniques. But while Steve seemed to be interested in his health, over the two years that I followed his progress in my office it became apparent that in spite of our efforts and his initial success, he slowly reverted to his previous habits. Two years after our last visit, I was informed he had suffered a second heart attack.

In a sense, both John and Steve approached their medical problems quite differently. John shifted responsibility for the care and treatment of his disease to the judgment and practices of his physicians, exclusively relying on drugs and surgery. In contrast, Steve began to use his own resources and capacities, practicing what we now call mind/body healing. But were their approaches really different? To an extent yes, but to a larger extent no. They both saw their heart disease as an abnormality to be fixed and treated. John applied conventional solutions to his problem, while Steve treated his problem with mind/body approaches. Both were exclusively motivated by the desire to avoid further illness and fix what was wrong. Surely we all would wish the same. Yet because both of these individuals viewed their lives through the perspectives of the treatment model, irrespective of the practices they used, they were unable to shift their focus from disease to health, and ultimately, neither of them could influence the course of their disease. Although their approaches may have differed—conventional versus mind/body—they were both exclusively focused on treatment, and so the results were the same.

What went wrong? Let's look at another case study. Marjorie, a successful attorney, also visited my office with advanced heart disease, and like Steve began to study and apply mind/body practices to the treatment of her illness. However, unlike John and Steve, Marjorie did not view the mind/body approaches she was learning as a form of treatment, but rather as an exciting new possibility for her life. She used the available pieces and parts of her life, her resources, capacities, newly acquired skills, *and the emotions and insights generated by her illness* to reshape her life and explore a different and more expansive way of living.

Over several years, through considerable effort, she developed an understanding of the sources of the conflicts and stresses in her life, expanded her relationships, experienced intimacy for the first time, trimmed her body weight, became an avid bicycler, and in her words, "began to appreciate the wonderful moments of everyday life." In this way the disease was integrated into her life, helping to provide character, meaning, direction, and enhanced resourcefulness, rather than shrinking and contracting her life until she "became" her disease. Marjorie had less and less use for my services as she continued to create a healthy way of living, one that served both to assist in the healing of her disease and to enhance the quality of her life. Could anyone doubt that she is a healthy woman in spite of her underlying disease?

Marjorie initially visited me to seek assistance with treating her disease using mind/body approaches. What she learned was far more valuable. She learned to seek health for its own sake. For her, health had value beyond its role in helping her recover from heart disease. If the heart disease was gone tomorrow, Marjorie would continue creating a healthy life. Initially her visit to me was motivated by the feelings of fear and deprivation resulting from her illness. Now she is motivated by the excitement, abundance, and possibilities generated by a healthy way of living. As important as it was to heal her disease, she was able to recognize that *health has value in and of itself.* She now knows that the presence of her disease did not exclude the possibility of health; in fact, in her case it provoked it. Health, she discovered, is a way we live our lives, a process that weaves through life's many seasons and is shaped by all of our experiences, disease included. Disease does not need to preclude health. It can, instead, awaken us to its possibilities.

COMPOSING A HEALTHY LIFE

In a sense, health is a creative process, one that is ongoing and changing throughout a lifetime. We take what we are given, "good" and "bad," and compose our lives of it. A healthy life is thus one of continual creation and re-creation. It is as if at each period of our lives we have a palette of colors with which we render the work of our lives. As our lives develop we add new colors. Sometimes these represent new insight and understanding, or recently developed skills and resources, and at times even adversity and disease. As the colors on our palette expand and change, our master work also changes. But at any time of life we can use what is given to us to compose and create the best possible work—one that explores all of the possibilities and potential that lie within the range of experiences that are given to us.

Over the period of a lifetime we will create many works, each of which will reflect the character and possibilities of the different stages of our lives. And in the end what will be of importance is that we have composed a life that was varied and full, one that included all of our possibilities and one that was aware and present at each moment of our creation. We will judge ourselves by the quality of our life rather than its longevity, by the success of our relationships rather than the balance in our bank account, and by our possibilities rather than our intermittent disabilities. This is a life of health, and, paradoxically, science is now demonstrating that it is also our best insurance against unnecessary disease. In this way, nature is economical. It gives us two for one.

THE QUALITIES
OF HEALTH

Greater than the treads of a mighty army is the power of an
idea whose time has come.

—Victor Hugo

The intention and direction of Whole Healing is fully realized
in the personal transformation that accompanies the expan
sion of consciousness and self-knowledge. This transformation is best seen in the appearance of certain personal
qualities, which seem to be clustered among those who exhibit
an unusual resistance to disease and an uncommon capacity
for full health. As we proceed successfully along the multi-
decade process of Whole Healing, we begin to acquire these
qualities, qualities that are the signposts indicating to us the
successful unfolding of the healing process. As we learn more
about the mechanisms of Whole Healing, it is becoming increasingly evident that these qualities are then translated,
through the neuropeptide messenger system, into physiological events that convey both the experience of hardiness and
the vitality of a fully lived life.

THE QUALITIES OF HEALTH

As a physician, I have had the extraordinary privilege of participating in the lives of my patients. In this process they have often related to me their life stories with complete candor and intimacy. I have heard the details of lives that have been exceptionally successful, and of others that have been marked by recurrent disappointment. Because of my interest in Whole Healing, I have listened with a certain ear, one that has sought to discern the distinguishing characteristics and qualities of those individuals who seem successful in their quest for health.

To expand this understanding further, I have turned to the work of those who have also carefully examined the qualities and characteristics of the healthy person. We have already seen the ideas of Aaron Antonovsky and Suzanne Kobassa, who both purport that psychological qualities can promote health and enhance our resistance to disease. To these I have added the work of Abraham Maslow and Carl Rogers, noted psychologists who studied and wrote about self-actualizing people, and Erik Erikson, a psychologist who offered us a detailed view of the healthy developmental process from childhood through adulthood.

In their work, a number of qualities that signaled health emerged. From these, seven characteristics of the healthy person, the qualities seen in the figure below, struck me as particularly important. Each of these qualities has many dimensions, and it is important to keep in mind that they develop to their fullest extent over many years. They provide us with both a resistance to disease and the potential to move toward full health and wholeness.

As I began to study and consider these qualities, I found myself assessing my own life, and in a sense taking an inventory of my progress in creating a healthy life. I was not so much measuring myself by a specific yardstick as inquiring into the areas on which I should place stronger emphasis. I reminded myself that this process is not linear and that each of these qualities continues to develop over a lifetime, relating in a synergistic manner to each of the other qualities. So I invite the reader to do the same: examine and explore your own development as we review each of the qualities of health.

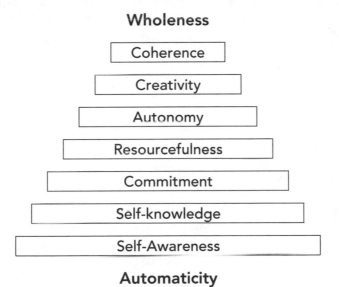

Wholeness

Coherence

Creativity

Autonomy

Resourcefulness

Commitment

Self-knowledge

Self-Awareness

Automaticity

These seven qualities can be considered the "signs and symptoms" of health. Each is built upon the preceding quality and provides the basis for the next quality.

During my workshops and in my work with individuals in the office, there often comes a time when we are able to sit quietly and share a very human conversation about life, and, more specifically, about the issues we are covering in this chapter. I have often been told that this relaxed dialogue is one of the more helpful and enriching experiences of our work together. Yet the issues we are about to discuss are complex, and each of us will likely explore them over many years. So take your time with this chapter, and perhaps even consider it a useful small primer in itself to come back to from time to time when one of these issues asserts itself in your life.

SELF-AWARENESS

The capacity for self-awareness is the underlying source from which all of the other qualities of health develop. Without it there is only a mechanical, programmed life. One must be able to look at life and see it directly before one can shift from the instinctual, automatic life that connects us to the animal kingdom to the consciousness and freedom that are both the source of health and our link to the spiritual.

I often begin my public lectures with a quotation, one that I have read so many times and in so many places that I can no longer remember the first time I encountered it. In its simplicity and directness it contains great power, a power that comes from the essential truths it conveys so well.

> Oh, I've had my moments, and if I had tried to do it over again, I'd have more of them. I'd try to have nothing else. Just moments, one after another, instead of living so many years ahead of each day.
>
> —Nadine Stair, age eighty-five

What does it mean to "have a moment"? For me it has come to mean the ability to experience a moment, to live in it fully aware, receptive, and appreciative of what is given. Whether the moment be one of pain, sorrow, or delight, it remains the only moment I have at that time. If I cannot experience it fully, then what moment am I experiencing? We know the answer all too well: We are occupied with yesterday, or tomorrow, one moment that is already gone, or another one that will likely be missed when it happens.

Self-awareness allows us to find our own path, our unique temperaments and capacities. In a way, it serves to deenculturate us. It helps us to see, and disempower, the many shoulds, shouldn'ts, and other perspectives that were instilled in us before we had the chance to choose for ourselves. It provides us with the opportunity to see people, things, and, most importantly, our own lives, as they are, without the shaping, defining, and constrictive effect of labels and conditioned interpretations. It brings a new freshness to each moment, an ability to see everything anew, from a different and changing perspective.

I would be foolish to suggest that self-awareness is a constant companion in our lives. It is not. The automatic mind is quite powerful and has a way of bringing us back to the inner dialogue. Yet I can now see the automatic mind for what it is, and although it has its roles, I am able to look at it, and gently move it aside. Never discarding it, for one cannot discard aspects of oneself, I simply recognize that it can be a valuable asset in my life when its actions are desirable and appropriate. But at other times it can be quite unhelpful. It is a part of me, but not all of me. It can serve me, but it does not need to overtake me.

As self-awareness has become a preferred way of being, I find myself calmer, clearer, more balanced, and more capable of understanding myself and my experiences. As this occurs, life seems easier, more natural, and less hurried. Everything gets done with more precision and heart, time seems to expand, I am more receptive and accepting of others, and, in general, my life seems more successful.

SELF-KNOWLEDGE

My sense is that the most important benefit I have received from self-awareness is the capacity to better understand myself and other people. What I first discovered was that it was actually possible to understand how my mind works. Over many years of self-exploration, I also learned that I was not one single being, but a complexity of parts: my acquired learning with its fixed perspectives and programs; my more natural and unique temperament, talents, and capacities; and my mind and body, which contain their own knowledge and wisdom. I was like an orchestra of many instruments requiring a conductor to direct the music.

But beyond ourselves is the important world of people and things, a world we are also meant to relate to. As we understand our past experiences and learn how to see ourselves and others without judging them according to our past, we become free to see life more clearly and act more appropriately, actions that will not leave us feeling angry, guilty, or resentful. When another person is angry it doesn't necessarily mean that we have done something wrong. We recognize that every individual interprets a situation according to his or her own perspective, and another person's anger may tell us more about his or her behavior than it tells us about our own. With self-knowledge, when it is important for us to say no, we can do so. We understand the inner voice that will avoid disapproval at any price, yet we can acknowledge it without acting on it. The same goes for saying yes. When we feel fearful or anxious we can look directly at its sources rather than running and distancing ourselves from experiences and people. Self-knowledge helps us to see what is without blaming ourselves or others, and if we wish to act in response to what we see, we can do so with clarity and directness.

I recognized that there were many potential sources to assist me in achieving self-knowledge. I have already mentioned the capacity of self-awareness to observe and discern the nature of one's own experience, and we have discussed the ability of people, things, our relationships, and life itself, to provide us with a mirror that can reflect back to us the aspects of ourselves that are either difficult to see or that we prefer not to see. I discovered, however, that underlying these teaching devices must be a basic philosophy of learning. One that has been most important to me is richly expressed in the teachings of J. Krishnamurti and C. G. Jung, who have both emphasized that when it comes to understanding or knowing oneself there can be no outer authority and no outer expert. To rely on another, at any level, is again to become enculturated, acquiring another set of views and expanding one's already overstocked memory with ideas that invariably belong to someone else, ideas containing the subjectivity and impressions specific to that individual's life experience. In Krishnamurti's words:

> Inquiry means hesitating, finding out for yourself, discovering step by step; and when you do that, then you need not follow anybody, you need not ask for correction or for confirmation of your discovery. But all this demands a great deal of intelligence and sensitivity. . . . The important thing is to discover, and after discovering, to keep going. It is detrimental to stay with what you have discovered, for then your mind is closed, finished. But if you die to what you have discovered the moment you have discovered it, then you can flow like the stream, like a river that has an abundance of water.

As I thought about these issues, I began to realize how much a part of my nature, and perhaps of all our natures, it has been to seek and gravitate toward those who "seem to know" in subtle and not so subtle ways, or even, as Krishnamurti has suggested, to hold on to my old viewpoints when they have become stale and outdated. Perhaps this is because it seems easier, or perhaps we have been taught not to trust our own capacities, our own wisdom. This may be the unfortunate side effect of an overemphasis on professionalism, which has in part developed at a cost to our lives. We have lost faith, respect, and the capacity to accomplish what we should do best: know ourselves.

Jung and Krishnamurti have written about the brilliant, inborn capacity for self-inquiry. They helped me to realize that all great thinkers and teachers rely on the same basic source for their knowledge and wisdom: *themselves*. The difference between their achievement and ours lies in their ability to listen to and trust their own experience and observations. We, in contrast, have been taught to listen to and trust others before ourselves. I am always amazed when individuals visit my office expecting that I could or should know more about their experience than they do. Not infrequently, such individuals have been living with symptoms for years, symptoms such as headaches, fatigue, and bowel disturbances, and yet they lack even the slightest understanding of the relationship between these symptoms and their life experience.

Self-knowledge grows as we begin to trust our experience and finely tune our capacity to observe it clearly. It requires that we begin to love the questions more than the answers. It demands our willingness to know that all of our knowledge, however accurate it may seem, is partial and always subject to revision. Yet the closer we get to the core of our experience, the more our knowledge resembles that of the great and wise thinkers. For the essential truths in life, although often expressed differently, come in a very few varieties. There is, however, a fundamental difference in arriving at the basic truths through one's own efforts in contrast to incorporating the views of others. In the first instance, we have fully developed our lives and taken in the truths that *we* have discovered; in the second circumstance we live a "secondhand," inauthentic life. We may know the correct answers, but we are unable to *live* them in our lives.

For me, there remains some comfort in the knowledge that there are mysteries and aspects of life that will likely remain unknowable and unnameable. Perhaps this is so because it denies me the opportunity to objectify life, and allows me to sustain a sense of awe at the magnitude and sacredness of what we each partake in. Beyond the knowing of myself, it is necessary for me to reflect upon the underlying forces that gave rise to and support the diversity of life, of which I am but one expression. And so I have discovered that on one hand it is essential for me to understand and live the life that is given to me, exactly as it is given, while on the other hand I realize that this specific and unique experience I call my life is part of a greater whole. Perhaps it is through the understanding of my local experience that I touch a larger sense of the underlying forces that sustain life.

COMMITMENT

A commitment is a pledge to which we bind ourselves. It could be to an ideal, a belief, a project, or a person. It is a choice to act in one way or another. It requires that we choose carefully among the many directions we can take in life. A commitment that arises from a firm self-knowledge and that expresses our unique values is necessarily an expression of self. This requires that we know ourselves, our values, our talents, and our deeply held convictions. In other words, a commitment does not arise from our minds and our thinking processes alone, but from the very fabric of our characters. In this sense it is natural rather than forced. It is as much a part of us as our feet and arms. Therefore to violate such a commitment is to violate ourselves.

What we give to our essential commitments is our life force. It is fair to ask, What do our commitments give to us? They help us to define our purpose, allowing us to come into relationship with experiences that convey value, importance, and sustaining interest. Commitments add meaning to our lives. Whether it is Viktor Frankl's commitment to bear his suffering so that he may survive to tell his story, my commitment to this writing, or your commitment to what holds value and meaning to you, commitment attaches itself to the things that have significance to us, and in turn deepens and focuses our energies. In this way commitment assists in defining the character of our lives.

It seems to me that the difficulty we have with commitment is our inability to recognize that it cannot be made meaningfully until we have reached a certain degree of self-understanding. Until then it is more likely to arise from our acquired shoulds and shouldn'ts, an action of our thoughts, rather than from our hearts and souls. The individual on the path to health who has approached his major life decisions through awareness and self-knowledge is able to make healthy and sustaining commitments that emerge from, and reflect, his or her nature. Such individuals are highly involved in their commitments, acting out of a sense of desire and delight rather than a sense of obligation and alienation.

Looking back, there were many years in my life when I could neither commit nor follow through on the few commitments I made. There was a sort of floundering, not knowing whether to go in this direction or that. It was not unusual for me to ask myself and my friends, "What do you think I should do?" I would try one thing and it wouldn't work, and then I'd try something else, and it also wouldn't seem right. I was putting the cart before the horse. I needed to back up a bit and change the question to "What are my nature and my character, my talents and my temperament? What is my particular 'song,' and how should I sing it?" Of course it took longer and considerably more effort to approach and explore these questions than deciding what to do in any particular instance. But as I became increasingly assured of the larger answers, the commitments came quickly and naturally. I discovered that I must observe and learn about my life and then allow the commitments that shape and give meaning to my existence to arise naturally from an understanding of myself. This does not mean that we should be immobilized until we have achieved some particular level of self-knowledge, but rather that until we feel a sense of confidence in our ability to sustain our commitments, we should approach them with care. And when they take us down the wrong road, we should learn from them and move on.

RESOURCEFULNESS

To be resourceful is to believe that you either have or can locate the skills, capacities, things, and people that are necessary

to meet the circumstances in your life. In a sense, resourcefulness is one end of a continuum, with helplessness at the other
end. Unlike the individual who responds to adversity by feeling
powerless, the resourceful individual meets the challenges of
life with enthusiasm, hopefulness, and confidence.

Resourcefulness implies a sense of inner control, an inner
certainty that one can influence the experience of one's life.
Such individuals look within to understand their experiences
and provide a meaning to them that supports the initiation of
positive and affirming actions. To do so, it is necessary to
make sense out of one's experiences, to be able to see them as
purposeful, meaningful, ordered, and necessary for the unfolding of one's life. This applies not only to the present, but also
to the past and future.

Resourcefulness implies a sense of initiative, a proactive
approach to life that is capable of forgetting past disappoint-
ments and energetically plans to undertake the next step in
life. In contrast to the outlook that sees life's events as being
random, chaotic, and lacking meaning (a viewpoint that underlies the experience of helplessness and powerlessness), the resourceful individual perceives the future with optimism, hope,
and trust. There is a strongly held feeling that one is responsible for one's life and has control over the attitudes and actions
that will ultimately define and shape it.

Resourcefulness is developmental. Early in life, its appearance is dependent on the demands presented by one's family.
If the demands are proportionate to our developing capacities,
we will learn that we can respond to life's circumstances effectively, challenging ourselves to extend our resources and to
develop new ones. If the demands upon us are excessive, we
will experience helplessness and frustration. If the demands
are insufficient, we will learn less in the way of initiative and
proactive action.

Later in life, when we are capable of defining our own lives,
developing and extending resourcefulness is a necessary activity of mind/body healing. We accomplish this by looking care-

fully at our lives, understanding our early childhood coding, and developing the skills, capacities, and resources necessary for an adult life. If it is not already present, we slowly gain a sense of confidence in our ability to manage our lives and meet the challenges presented to us.

AUTONOMY

Autonomy is the acceptance of responsibility for the authorship and governance of one's life. It reflects a basic trust in one's capacity to understand life and its experiences, and a confidence that one can find, irrespective of the circumstance, the resources and capacities to manage life. There is no room here for the "pointing finger" or the endless rationalizations. My life is my life. It can be lived only once and must be lived according to my temperament, capacities, values, and beliefs. It is necessary that I make the best of whatever I am given, or, as it is said, whatever hand I draw. I am interdependent, but not dependent. I have needs, but also the resources to meet them.

Autonomy must not be mistaken for what is commonly referred to as independence, particularly the loudly proclaimed type of independence, which is more likely a counterbalancing reaction to a deeply felt dependence. It is not measured by the number of things I can do for myself, or my capacity to be separate from others. It is an inner attitude based on a process of psychological development that quietly, maturely, and in unassuming ways accepts the reality of self-responsibility. Paradoxically, it is these individuals who are most capable of surrendering themselves into intimacy, work, or service. Unlike those who profess an inauthentic "independence," autonomous individuals know that despite the circumstances of one's life it is not possible to lose one's basic identity any more than it is possible to lose one's body.

Autonomy completes a circle that begins with the necessity of the infant to trust others, and ends with the necessity of the adult to trust him- or herself. As the infant is dependent on the skills and resources of its parents, the adult is similarly dependent on his or her own skills and resources. Whereas it is the environment of the child that determines his development, it is the initiative and intention of the adult that defines the ultimate character of his or her life. Autonomy is the fully realized capacity to orchestrate one's life.

CREATIVITY

Creativity, the capacity for originality and inventiveness, is the result of the ability to perceive experiences in a fresh, uninhibited, and penetrating way. Unlike the special talents and gifts that seem to come with birth to the creative genius, this capacity is developed over time. In a sense, it is a return by the mature, healthy adult to the spontaneity and natural creativity of the child, a creativity that is often suppressed with the development of self-consciousness.

Creativity is very much linked to the expansion of consciousness. As the conditioned mind can only produce thoughts, feelings, and images that are old, originality is not one of its resident characteristics. Only the capacity to let go of automatic thinking and activate present-moment awareness can unleash the potential for creativity. Lacking a sense of time or memory and incapable of placing old meanings on new experiences, full awareness provides the context for creativity.

Creativity can be applied to all aspects of life. Cooking dinner, preparing clothes, building a cabinet, and interacting with people are just a few examples. It is a certain attitude and spirit, a certain optimism, spontaneity, and delight, which infuses all of an individual's experiences with a sense of freshness, simplicity, and directness. Each day and each moment of life are available as new experiences and new possibilities. Each experience is another opportunity to discover people and things anew.

Creativity can also be structured. It is a subtle process that first requires the capacity to stabilize the mind in silence. In silence, it is possible to pose a problem to the mind, and, avoiding the tendency to analyze it through one's intellect, allow intuitive thinking to provide an original solution, one that is not shaped by the conditioned mind. Actually, I think we often do this naturally, and when we do, we can recognize it by the appearance of a spontaneous insight, an "aha" experience. Perhaps we naturally seek silence at the beach or in the mountains because it assists us with unfolding new approaches to old problems. It is quite possible that with the development of consciousness we can learn to turn on and direct creativity at will.

As a physician, I would like to think that beyond our aesthetic and problemsolving creative talents, we are also capable of working creatively with our physiology. The work in PNI, as we discussed previously, suggests that as we alter our mental life we also alter our physiology, and we are quite aware, as we have discussed, of the ways we can enhance our resistance to disease and assist in recovery by developing our Mind/Body Healing System. If we look at some of the more unusual conscious acts of self-regulation (for example, the capacity to walk on hot coals, the capacity of Yogis to remain buried for days without oxygen, or the capacity to stop bleeding through conscious intention) one wonders how far we can go with effort and creativity in affecting our physiology.

In a sense, the entire process of health and healing is a creative act. For most of us, and more specifically for our culture, health and healing as we have spoken of them comprise a fresh, original and inventive response to our lives, one that stands separate and distinct from customary ideas about health and disease.

COHERENCE

A sense of coherence emerges with the development of the preceding qualities of health: self-awareness, self-knowledge, commitment, resourcefulness, autonomy, and creativity. It doesn't come all at once. Rather, it slowly arises as we grow and mature into our lives. It is a progressive coming together of knowledge, resources, capacities, confidence, and competence. At first coherence may last for only a few fleeting moments, and perhaps it will still be somewhat dependent on outer circumstances. Eventually it persists for longer periods and it is less reliant on external support. It brings with it feelings of optimism and confidence, an understanding of one's place in the world, and a remarkable sense of ease and comfort. Motivation arises from within, and gratification results from a personal sense of achievement rather than social applause.

In my own life, I have watched this develop very slowly over time, and have noticed that the capacity to experience coherence developed in parallel with a discovery of my natural directions, allowing me to experience passion and certainty in both my short- and long-term choices. Coherence is achieved by living life in accordance with one's nature, as Nietzsche said, "Become what thou art." It is then possible to do one's best in a manner that is consistent with oneself. In this instance the outer life is seen to be in direct continuity with the inner life.

"So," my patients ask me, "how do I find out what I'm supposed to do with my life so I can get on with it and do my life's work?" Of course I cannot answer this question directly. To try to do so is to succumb to the mentality of the traditional treatment method of healing, to belief in the magic bullet. What I can do is point out that an understanding of oneself and one's natural inclinations in life cannot be arrived at by any means other than the effort required in achieving health through Whole Healing—the process we have been examining in this book—and the qualities that evolve from these efforts. What can be said is that even when we start with an intent as simple as paying attention to our day-to-day lives, something happens that is new and fresh. Perhaps we will discover that we are on the wrong track and need to explore another option, or we may discover that we have chosen the correct course. If we continue to pay attention to our lives, listening carefully to how our bodies respond to our choices, we will be continuously learning about ourselves. Each activity and each commitment can bring more understanding and clarity. It is important to remember that coherence is not a problem to be solved, but rather the result of a consciously considered life.

This must be contrasted with the individual—and we have all seen many of them—who appears to know everything and exude a somewhat rigid self-assurance. Such an individual has replaced personal development and the qualities we have discussed with a borrowed set of values and beliefs. Although it is possible for such individuals to navigate quite successfully within the narrow bounds of their subculture, this inauthentic sense of coherence is quite vulnerable and rapidly breaks down if the individual attempts to live outside of the boundaries of his or her particular belief system. I often see highly successful businesspeople whose confidence and competence in the business environment seems strangely incompatible with their unhealthy personal lives, which require very different personal qualities, ones that must be developed rather than borrowed. The individual who has developed coherence from the inside out exudes a sense of self that is enduring and invulnerable. It applies to outer circumstances as well as inner ones.

A fully developed sense of coherence is the mark of a fully developed Mind/Body Healing System. It rests upon the assimilation and mastery of the capacity for silence, self-inquiry, and intuitive insight. There is a sense of self that comes with coherence that is *difficult to define in words*. Perhaps this is because it is sufficiently uncommon that the words would be unfamiliar. The best we can do is to recall those moments in life when we felt most balanced, centered, easeful, confident, and effective. It is as if one is standing tall and straight, meeting the world with delight, assurance, and competence. For most, this is a fleeting experience, but for those who have persistently pursued Whole Healing this becomes a more regular, and, finally, a permanent part of life.

Related Attributes

Healthy people often live within a culture in which the qualities of health are rare. For this individual there is an ongoing negotiation between his or her knowledge, autonomy, creativeness, and values, and the realities of society. There are various resolutions to this dilemma. Some individuals may use their insight and understandings to work in society in very practical ways, facilitating social change where it is possible. Others may keep to themselves. These individuals are often artists, poets, or writers. Still others commit their lives to compassionate service. And there are yet those who never quite resolve this problem. They are uncomfortable in a world of greed, unnecessary poverty, and hypocrisy, yet they have neither found a way to accept what is and work for change within the structure of society, nor are they comfortable with a life that lives on the margins of the cultural experience. The resulting tension must be used as an impetus for yet further development and understanding, the only alternative being despair.

Healthy individuals also have a desire and need for solitude. They are at peace alone. Solitude allows them to "feel" their lives, enjoy the simple pleasures of life, and avoid and recover from the endless chatter and stresses of an anxious and unhealthy society. At times, much as is the experience of the introvert, this desire to be alone can be misunderstood as unfriendly and uncaring, but it is not. In fact, such individuals have very deep friendships, although these are limited to individuals whose life experiences make it possible to understand the character and nature of the healthy life.

Finally, those who have actively pursued the qualities of health are able, with an increasing frequency, to experience wholeness. This experience is most commonly present in individuals who have "grown" their health. It is not only peace, harmony, and joy that are found, but also the extraordinary perspective and insight into self and others that is gained from the transcendent perspective of wholeness. There is a personal and somewhat mystical experience of the unifying forces of life, one that forever shifts and changes how we see and experience our lives.

I wish I could say that there is a large body of research that can further inform us about the character and quality of health and Whole Healing, but there is not. We still live within a framework that is entranced with disease, its diagnoses, pathogenesis, and treatment. Ironically, we have mastered a science of disease, but lack even the rudiments of a science of health.

Antonovsky, Kobassa, and other researchers we have discussed earlier in this book have helped to describe the personal qualities that provide an active resistance to disease. Although this is a part of our goal, we are also concerned about the movement toward wholeness, which in our view is the fulfillment of health. For this we must look toward others. Jung, Maslow, and other modern-day developmental psychologists have attempted to begin the exploration of these issues. They have provided us with guidance and direction regarding them.

Meanwhile, we are indeed fortunate that nature, which is both economical and efficient (these are again Jung's words), has provided us with a unified path, one that we have called Whole Healing, which results in the development of the qualities that simultaneously convey a resistance to disease and lead us toward wholeness. This is as it should be. The more one studies life, the more apparent it is that in spite of our need to tamper with it, nature has a brilliance that is unmatched by human endeavor; and yet at the same time, as a part of nature, if we would only listen we may also discover our own brilliance.

ORCHESTRATING
HEALTH

The most beautiful and deepest experience a man can have is
the sense of the mysterious. It is the underlying principle of
religion as well as of serious endeavors in art and science.
—Albert Einstein

We are coming of age, and in matters of health we now have
the capacity, even given the highly technical nature of medicine, to orchestrate our personal health, that is, to compose,
organize, coordinate, manage, and integrate all of our health-
related efforts. This does not require that we become technical
experts, or that our judgment be as developed as that of a professional. Nor does it require a specialized expertise similar to
that of a trained practitioner. Instead it requires expertise in
managing our health needs: understanding the values we hold
concerning health, our healing capacities, our ability to use
each of the healing systems as needed, the capacity to access
up-to-date information on the many approaches to healing,
and a willingness to reappropriate our central and essential
role in decisions that concern our health.

WHAT WE BELIEVE

When it comes to our health what we believe is what we get. Whole Healing requires a set of attitudes that have not as yet been widely considered in our culture. Here are some essential values that underlie these attitudes and Whole Health:

1. *Health is an active process.* Health is not a part of life that sits on a shelf separated from the rest of our experience, or in a drawer that we open only when we become ill. It is an ongoing active process that moves us progressively toward a fully integrated sense of self—what we have called wholeness. When we choose a profession, we study and practice the principles and art of that profession. Health is no different. It requires study and practice, study of ourselves, study of life, and then the lifelong practice of healthy living. We are not taught this in school; therefore it must be self-taught.

2. *Health is possible even in adversity.* Health is a way of living characterized by awareness, knowledge, and wholeness. It requires that adversity be seen as a challenge and an opportunity, a message that assists us in defining the next movement in our lives, urging us to expand our consciousness and become larger than we have been. Disease is an aspect of the living experience. It does not define our state of health: What does define our state of health is how we approach it. This is not an easy issue for anyone to grasp. Wilfred Sheed, whose book *In Love with Daylight* relates his battle with polio, addictions, and cancer, states it this way: "One man's wonderful challenge and chance to defy the gods is made of the same substance as another man's sweat-drenching nightmare."

3. *Health has many faces.* We have learned from the four healing systems that health is more than one thing. It is the natural balancing and self-healing of the homeostatic system, the restoration of function that can be accomplished through the treatment system, the growth of consciousness that characterizes the mind/body system, and the achievement of

wholeness and spirituality. Although we may be oriented toward Whole Health, at any one moment we may focus on one or another aspect of healing: learning to consider adversity as a challenge and opportunity, learning to use the treatment system effectively and confidently, mastering the capacity for intimacy, becoming comfortable with time alone, committing ourselves to the development of consciousness, and, in time, discovering the aesthetic and the spiritual. Life provides us with lessons and challenges that assist us as we traverse the specific issues of each of its seasons. It is not possible for us to organize the flow of life; for health we must use what is given to us and learn and grow from these experiences.

4. *We are the authors of our health.* No person, practice, theory, or institution can make us healthy. It is ultimately something we can do only for ourselves. This is a difficult task to take on in the face of the many practices, services, or products promising health. If, as we have come to believe as a culture, the treatment system and its unchallenged authority is the only path to healing, then there is no choice. But we know we have larger possibilities. To activate these we must be willing to shift our worldview, recognizing in that revolutionary act that we can now see who and what we are. With that vision we can become more than we have ever been, authors of our own experience and cocreators with evolution.

5. *We contain within us the wisdom we need to be healthy.* I have often said to my clients that the only thing that separates any one of us from the great sages is that they know how to listen to the mind and body, to learn from life itself. We don't use this ability, though we have the same material to work with as they did. Encoded in our minds and bodies is the entire wisdom of the millennia of human development. This is why in my office practice, I try to listen to my clients, and to the message that is concealed in the presenting symptoms. Listening is a skill we can develop, and the more we listen the more we understand and live in concert with life rather than in opposition to it.

USING OUR HEALING SYSTEMS

Understanding our values about health underlies the way we proceed to orchestrate our health. The first part of the program is that we accept values that are consistent with health; when we do so, we become capable of the next step, understanding and using the healing systems available to each of us. We have discussed these in detail in the preceding chapters, but I would like to return to them once more to clarify the specific steps that are necessary to activate each system fully. You can refer to the chart on the next page for a handy summary of the four healing systems.

THE HOMEOSTATIC READING SYSTEM

The central characteristic of this system is its capacity for self-healing. The central task for users of this system is to learn to "listen" to the body with sufficient care to "hear" its needs. This system requires that we heed the nonverbal information provided to us by the body. When we listen we will know when we are out of balance, and what is required to restore the conditions under which our body can rebalance itself. When we don't listen we will learn of imbalance in its more overt forms, the signs and symptoms of disease. Stay "in touch" with this system; it is the most profound and fundamental healing system available to us.

THE TREATMENT HEALING SYSTEM

The central characteristic of the treatment healing system is the use, usually by practitioners, of external agents to manipulate the mind and body for the purpose of repairing abnormalities and restoring normal function. The task for users of this system is to become knowledgeable about its various options so as to be able to make informed choices. When we

The Four Healing Systems

SYSTEM	CHARACTERISTIC	CENTRAL TASK FOR USERS
Homeostatic	Knowledge of and capacity for self-healing	Learning to listen to the body to hear its needs
Treatment	Use of external agents to manipulate mind and body for the purpose of repairing abnormalities and restoring normal function	Becoming knowledgeable about the system's options in order to make informed choices
Mind/Body	Activates self-regulation and self-exploration	Self-inquiry
Spiritual	The capacity to reorganize and harmonize psychology and physiology holistically	Discovering meaning and wholeness

think of treatment we usually think of the biomedical system and its use of drugs and surgery. But most alternative therapies, for example, chiropractic, acupuncture, homeopathy, Ayurvedic, energy transfer, body work, and so on, are, as generally practiced, also treatments. Some alternative therapies may be more risk free or more broadly based than others, but in practice they remain something done to us by a professional through the use of an external agent.

There is a place for treatment and a legitimate reason to seek more choices than we currently have. To use this system appropriately we must be willing to commit ourselves to the task of gathering information on the various treatment systems to determine both efficacy and potential side effects. Treatment is never a substitute for personal growth, or the development and use of our inner resources. But there will always be a time when treatment, when used with care, knowledge, and appropriateness, has its place in an overall program of recovery. Please remember that treatment is always a reactive rather than a proactive activity and as such is used not to maintain health, but as one possible resource when health has failed.

THE MIND/BODY HEALING SYSTEM

Our first sense of mind/body healing is that it is a way we use the mind to heal the body. Of course this is true, but this system has a second aspect—self-exploration. This aspect focuses on the intentional expansion of consciousness and the attainment of self-knowledge and autonomy. It requires a certain degree of silence and a commitment to self-inquiry. When we expand consciousness we heal attitudes and perspectives, which in turn leads to a healing of our physiology, a natural and more permanent self-regulation. We seek to acquire the qualities of health, the attitudes and capacities that are consistent with a healthy life. This is a lifetime commitment to composing a vital and creative life, a commitment to studying, to attending seminars and workshops or other activities that stimulate the expansion of consciousness. And it most surely means ongoing self-questioning.

THE SPIRITUAL HEALING SYSTEM

There are two aspects to spiritual healing: the discovery of meaning and the experience of wholeness. Meaning reorganizes and harmonizes our psychology and physiology. Whether we are speaking about the discovery of meaning in our daily lives or in our relatedness to nature, spiritual healing can emerge from, but does not require, the form and structure of an organized faith. It does require staying in touch with the messages and guidance we receive from our lives, and simultaneously staying in touch with the voice of the spirit. When one is open and available to the simplicity and clarity of each moment, spirituality is present.

The figure below shows us the four interactive components of the Whole Healing System. As we discussed in Chapter 1, this complete system, taken as a whole, provides us with a natural, living healing system. Any individual component, taken by itself, cannot sustain us in mind and body. The parts are essential to the whole, and the whole is essential to the parts.

THE INTERACTIVE AND INTEGRATED HEALING SYSTEM

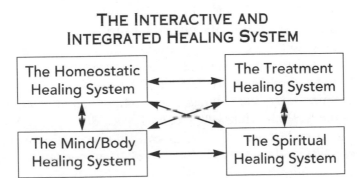

The four healing systems are interactive with each other at all times. Having said this, it must also be remembered that in life they are not four, but one.

ADAPTING THE MODEL TO OUR
LIFE CIRCUMSTANCES

The way we use the various capacities of our healing system depends upon the circumstances of our lives. How we start and where we start is determined by several factors. If we wait until we are ill, which unfortunately seems to be our inclination, we will likely start with the treatment system. If the problem is an acute and short-lived one, we will usually avail ourselves of the customary treatments, recover shortly, and return to life as usual. If the problem is of a more chronic nature, recurrent, or serious, we should look beyond the limitations of the Treatment Healing System and any other one-treatment approach.

Let's review what happens in each of these instances. A cold, a muscle strain, a skin rash, or a host of other minor problems usually call for caring, rest, and perhaps treatment of one form or another. Even in these instances it is fair to ask ourselves whether an intensification of stress at work or at home, poor eating or sleep habits, or a lack of exercise, conditions that are inconsistent with the natural healing efforts of the homeostatic system, have preceded the onset of illness. Here is a typical exchange: "I've had this cold for two weeks and it won't go away." My questions are always the same, "How many hours a week are you working? How are things at home? How are you eating and exercising? And, have you listened to your body and taken time off to rest?" The answer is usually something like: "Things are on a tight schedule at work so I've not had any time off." Again I ask, "How many hours did you work last week?" The answer is usually somewhere between fifty and seventy (I always add 10 percent to the estimate).

The point is that even with a minor self-resolving problem it is important for each of us to see the connection between the way we live our lives and the development of disease. So orchestrating the care of such a problem can inform us about the way we support or undermine our natural healing capacities, and how our attitudes and perspectives can set us up for illness. Even a minor illness can encourage us to seek out different approaches to treatment, a process that sets us on the path of learning about the multitude of treatment options that may be available to us for future use.

A recurrent, chronic, or serious problem calls upon us to understand and use each of the healing systems and, when it comes to the treatment system, to broaden our choices to consider various treatment approaches. The first step must always be to care for any acute problems that require immediate intervention. Usually this occurs through biomedicine, which generally does quite well with emergency care. It is my experience that in such circumstances alternative practitioners will usually defer to biomedicine, an indication of their flexibility and capability of working within a multiapproach framework—something many physicians have yet to learn. But once the acute care is accomplished, there are many further decisions to be made. Physicians do not have a monopoly on making the next set of choices—we do. The questions to ask include:

- Considering the *homeostatic system*—How can I support my natural healing systems? Rest, food, exercise, attitudes, social support and nurturing, a change in surroundings?

- Considering the *treatment system*—What are the best treatment approaches to this problem, their efficacy and side effects? Where can I find the information I need to evaluate them?

- Considering the *mind/body system*—What does this disruption tell me about the way I have been living my life, my habits, attitudes, and environment? What personal qualities must I draw upon and develop to enhance recovery and my future well-being? How can I use my mind to assist with healing my body?

- Considering the *spiritual system*—How can I find a meaning, purpose, and significance in the adversity I am living through? Why this illness, why me, and why now?

- Considering the *Whole Healing System*—If I was composing my life as if it were one great work of art, how would I do it and what would it look like?

For someone unfamiliar with an expanded approach to healing, it is necessary first to find good, up-to-date sources of information (specific suggestions are provided in the resources section). It may also be helpful to find a guide, a person who can challenge you with questions, suggest readings, seminars, and workshops, and help to expand your perspectives. The shift from the acute phase of an illness to its chronic phase is a shift of responsibility from the practitioner to the individual. Chronic and recurrent disease is a wake-up call urging us on to a richer and fuller understanding of our life and of living itself.

THE WHOLE HEALING SYSTEM AT WORK

Let's now look at how the Whole Healing System can apply all of its resources to one of the most urgent and difficult problems of daily life: stress. Each healing system will respond in a different way. In isolation, these separate responses would be less effective, but when organized as a coherent whole, the coordinated response to stress results in the development of new skills and resources and serves the purpose of insuring survival, and promoting growth and revitalization.

The homeostatic system experiences stress as a disruption to the normal steady-state conditions of the mind and body. This system automatically activates the stress response to prepare the body to cope with danger, and then just as rapidly shuts down the response as soon as the danger has passed. The treatment system experiences stress and its direct physiological consequences as problems to be solved, usually through the use of drugs to treat its secondary effects, including headaches, ulcers, colitis, anxiety, and musculoskeletal disorders. In the Mind/Body Healing System, stress is seen as an opportunity to develop and apply self-regulation skills, and as a source of growth, change, and healing. The Spiritual Healing System views unrelenting stress as a message that suggests a reconsideration of one's fundamental outlook on life, an intimation of a renewed search for meaning and purpose. It is seen as a profound statement that informs us that it is time to re-examine our lives, grow, and change.

Together, the four healing systems contribute to a fully integrated response to stress.

THE RESPONSE TO STRESS: THE HOMEOSTATIC HEALING SYSTEM

The Homeostatic Healing System responds to stress through the automatic activation of emotional and physical protective mechanisms. This response evolved as a means of insuring survival by activating the mind and body for vigilance and rapid action, thereby protecting us from imminent physical threat or danger. The major contribution of this system is its capacity for immediate action, an immediacy that can be lifesaving when we are confronted with a sudden threat to our survival, a circumstance that may not allow for the luxury of the time that is required for conscious deliberation. The natural tendency of the homeostatic response is to turn itself off as soon as the immediacy of the danger has receded. It is designed as a rapid "on and off" response to physical danger.

THE IMMEDIATE PHYSICAL RESPONSE TO STRESS

Redirection of body nutrients to the brain and stressed body sites
Increased blood pressure and heart rate
Increased respiratory rate
Increased glucose production and fat breakdown for quick energy
Inhibition of growth and reproductive systems

THE IMMEDIATE EMOTIONAL RESPONSE TO STRESS

Increased arousal, alertness
Increased cognition, vigilance
Focused attention
Decrease in nonadaptive behaviors (eating, sexuality)

But while these responses once served a useful purpose by alerting us to danger, despite the best efforts of our Homeostatic Healing System, it is unprepared to resolve the character, intensity, and persuasiveness of the stresses of today's urban life.

THE RESPONSE TO STRESS: THE TREATMENT HEALING SYSTEM

The stress that we confront today is very different from the threat of imminent physical danger for which the Homeostatic Healing System evolved. We suffer from unrelenting mental stress, which is chronic rather than intermittent, and most often is imagined rather than real physical danger. Because we cannot get away from stress, the homeostatic system remains continuously activated, maintaining our minds and bodies in an ongoing protective and defensive mode, a deadly distortion of the direction and intent of the Homeostatic Healing System. We are so accustomed to chronic stress that we rarely identify its presence, as it masquerades as "normal." We are similarly unaware of its long-term impact, failing to recognize the symptoms of chronic disease from their association with years of chronic stress. In fact, few of us know what it feels like for the stress response to shut down. What we consider to be relaxation is usually simply our lowest level of stress.

The inability of the homeostatic system to respond successfully to chronic stress drives us to develop ways to treat the consequences of unrelenting stress. For this we have invented a variety of treatments (for example, medications for anxiety, stomach distress, headaches, and insomnia), which can diminish the overt consequences of chronic stress. To some extent these treatments may lessen symptoms, which can be an important contribution to the overall healing of stress. But treatment most often provides a false sense of optimism and fails to distinguish the difference between treating symptoms and healing the source of the problem. As an isolated approach to stress, treatment can also be counterproductive, as its tendency to lessen overt symptoms "covers up" the more fundamental questions raised by the appearance of stress. Recently a friend of mine who is a psychiatrist described to me his attempt to use medications, in this instance the antidepressant Prozac, to relieve disabling feelings of anxiety and depression, highlighting this dilemma. "Prozac allowed me to function again," he said. "It allowed me to keep my hand in the fire *far longer than I should have*."

Because it exclusively relies on external resources, the Treatment Healing System is designed only to allay the symptoms of stress: It fails to prompt us to reconsider our attitudes and lifestyles, two important sources of stress.

THE RESPONSE TO STRESS: THE MIND/BODY HEALING SYSTEM

The Mind/Body Healing System can play an important role in the resolution of stress. If they are activated by the individual, its two components, self-regulation and self-exploration, will achieve the dual role of providing skills that can immediately reduce stress levels and furnish the self-knowledge that can lead to attitude and lifestyle change, which will convey a future resistance to stress.

When we apply self-regulation skills to the alleviation of stress, they actually serve two purposes. First, as mentioned above, these practices (many of which we have already discussed in this chapter) can relieve the immediate symptoms of stress, diminishing the need for drugs, other treatments, and their unwanted side effects. Second, rather than feeling dependent on such aids, we are empowered with a new self-reliant way of handling stress, practices that we can apply by ourselves whenever we need to. I cannot emphasize how important it is for an individual to feel confident that he or she has the resources to respond to life's stresses effectively. This knowledge alone can serve to enhance an individual's resistance to stress.

If we are motivated by the presence of stress to activate the second component of mind/body healing, self-exploration, we are sure to learn about the sources of stress in our lives and consider the necessary changes in attitudes and lifestyles that will guarantee a less conflicted life. Exploring stress in this manner can lead to the type of self-knowledge that can guide us in very new directions. We may discover that certain circumstances of our lives need modification. We may find that our past experiences, experiences that often intensify stress by interpreting current events as threatening, need to be understood and left in the past. Our relationships may need work, or we may need to reexamine our work situation. When we fully apply the Mind/Body Healing System to the issue of stress, stress becomes an important opportunity to learn and grow.

THE RESPONSE TO STRESS:
THE SPIRITUAL HEALING SYSTEM

The Spiritual Healing System seeks meaning in our day-to-day experiences, and simultaneously offers a larger vision of life, one that will in itself change the way we respond to people and things. We all know that when we are in the presence of the great events of life, those problems that always appear so large become smaller, assigning to themselves a more appropriate place in the order of things. With this spiritual perspective we can turn what has been perceived as a dangerous and threatening circumstance into a more minor event, neutralizing the potential for stress. And when excessive stress is present, the spiritual perspective can see its meaning and purpose at that particular moment in life. This viewpoint turns the situation around, from one that is negative and to be avoided to one that needs to be understood, confronted and ultimately viewed from a wider angle.

For all of its unpleasantness, we can now understand that stress, when properly understood and explored, may be preferable to a life that seems oblivious to stress. In the latter instance, individuals may avoid the suffering involved, but they will simultaneously lose an important force in life, a force that can serve to motivate, initiate, and activate the Whole Healing process. It is only when stress is seen from the perspective of *dynamism, holism,* and *purposefulness,* the assumptions of the Whole Healing System, that it becomes an integral part of the process of growing and healing our lives.

Our examination of stress has allowed us to see how the four healing systems are integrated in response to distress, but the Whole Healing model is appropriate to all of life's physical and mental ills. The point is to understand the roles of the four aspects of Whole Healing, and that they are always available to us.

The commitment to health and healing is a lifelong process. To approach our own health proactively, not requiring ourselves to become sick in order to motivate ourselves toward health, is the act of a maturing mind. It is unusual for me to meet a truly healthy individual in my practice (this is as it should be). When I do, they are usually reading books, attending seminars, experimenting with life, and always growing and changing in new directions. For them disease is a challenge, directing them toward the exploration of a new set of ideas and issues. These are vital people whose awareness is growing, whose resources and capacities are increasingly more varied, and who are clearly claiming ownership and authorship of their lives. Careful listening informs them about the status of the homeostatic system, analytical research and empirical evidence feed their knowledge of the treatment system, psychosocial information and self-inquiry expand their understanding of the mind/body system, and a conscious movement through the existential issues of life opens up their spiritual capacity. For them, recovery, health, autonomy, and wholeness are the results of a self-orchestrated healing process.

Just as a composer must know the range and capacities of each instrument and musician, so must we know the range of capacities of each of our healing systems. I have provided you with an overview of your healing capacities. The appendix will assist you with a reading list and advice on topical periodicals, and will offer a resource guide. These will help you fill in the details and take the next step as you begin this lifelong journey toward autonomy, health, and wholeness.

∽

INNER JOURNEY #8:
SURVEYING THE HEALING SYSTEMS

This exercise will assist you in attaining more fluency with the issues involved in each of the healing systems. Consider it a tool for awareness that you can use whenever it is needed.

THE HOMEOSTATIC HEALING SYSTEM

	Sometimes	Always	Never
1. Are you aware of and do you believe in the connection between how you live your life and your state of health?	☐	☐	☐

	Sometimes	Always	Never
2. Do you use preventive strategies, for example, nonsmoking, exercise, healthy eating, flossing, safely belts?	☐	☐	☐
3. Do you feel rested when you arise in the morning?	☐	☐	☐
4. Do you have plenty of energy?	☐	☐	☐
5. Do you take time to rest when fatigued, time to heal when sick, and time to relax when stressed?	☐	☐	☐
6. Are you aware of how your physical environments affect your well-being?	☐	☐	☐
7. Do you avoid unhealthy environments?	☐	☐	☐
8. Do you nurture yourself?	☐	☐	☐
9. Are you aware of the effects of different foods on your mind and body?	☐	☐	☐
10. Are you aware of the effect of healthy relationships on your mind and body?	☐	☐	☐
11. Are you aware of the subtle messages from your mind and body?	☐	☐	☐
12. Are you aware of subtle changes in your mind and body?	☐	☐	☐
13. Are you aware of how to use your natural healing capacities?	☐	☐	☐
14. Do you adjust your life to respond to the needs of your mind and body?	☐	☐	☐
15. Do you think of your natural healing capacities before treatment?	☐	☐	☐

THE TREATMENT HEALING SYSTEM

	Sometimes	Always	Never
1. Do you consider all of the treatment systems available to you?	☐	☐	☐
2. Do you feel competent to judge the effectiveness of the treatment system you are using?	☐	☐	☐
3. Do you feel informed about the available options?	☐	☐	☐
4. Are you comfortable with professionals?	☐	☐	☐
5. Do you exclusively rely on the treatment system?	☐	☐	☐
6. Do you feel that treatment systems are the best way to cure disease?	☐	☐	☐
7. Do you think of treatment in terms of fixing and repairing?	☐	☐	☐
8. Do you think of treatment in terms of growth? In terms of change?	☐	☐	☐
9. Do you often consider a professional your main source of healing?	☐	☐	☐
10. Are you satisfied when you are feeling "normal"?	☐	☐	☐
11. Do you feel in charge when you are receiving treatment?	☐	☐	☐

THE MIND/BODY HEALING SYSTEM

	Sometimes	Always	Never
1. Do you feel passion in your life?	☐	☐	☐
2. Do problems seem like challenges and opportunities?	☐	☐	☐
3. Do you feel powerless and victimized?	☐	☐	☐

	Sometimes	Always	Never
4. Are your feelings and thoughts confused, conflictual, and worrisome?	☐	☐	☐
5. Do you feel comfortable being alone?	☐	☐	☐
6. Do you feel comfortable with intimacy?	☐	☐	☐
7. Do you use drugs, relationships, or possessions to avoid difficult feelings?	☐	☐	☐
8. Do you get busy as a way of avoiding difficult feelings?	☐	☐	☐
9. Do you regularly have thoughts or feelings you would prefer to avoid?	☐	☐	☐
10. Are you aware of the mind's effect on the body and the body's effect on the mind?	☐	☐	☐
11. Do you feel autonomous and self-sufficient?	☐	☐	☐
12. Do you feel creative?	☐	☐	☐
13. Do you feel you can find answers to most problems?	☐	☐	☐
14. Do you feel that life can always be managed?	☐	☐	☐
15. Do you react automatically to events rather than doing what is truest to your own beliefs and goals?	☐	☐	☐
16. Do you believe that health is an ongoing proactive experience rather than an accident of fortune?	☐	☐	☐

THE SPIRITUAL HEALING SYSTEM

	Sometimes	Always	Never
1. Do you feel a lack of concern about things that happen around you?	☐	☐	☐
2. Do you find life interesting and adventurous?	☐	☐	☐

	Sometimes	Always	Never
3. Do you feel that things rarely make sense?	☐	☐	☐
4. Do your day-to-day activities have meaning and purpose?	☐	☐	☐
5. Do you feel that life in the future will be meaningful and purposeful?	☐	☐	☐
6. Do you experience a connection among the diverse aspects of life?	☐	☐	☐
7. Do you feel a oneness and unity with life?	☐	☐	☐
8. Do you experience synchronistic events in your life?	☐	☐	☐
9. Does the idea of the divine have a particular meaning to you?	☐	☐	☐
10. Do you have a sense of having enough?	☐	☐	☐
11. Do you trust nonverbal, noncognitive ways of knowing?	☐	☐	☐
12. Do you feel a sense of awe and wonder about life?	☐	☐	☐
13. Are you comfortable with the mysterious aspects of life?	☐	☐	☐
14. Can you feel the healing effects of a spiritual perspective?	☐	☐	☐

There is no score to this survey. The idea is to stimulate your thinking and help you to identify areas you may wish to change.

∽

INNER JOURNEY # 9:
STRESS AS TEACHER, STRESS AS HEALER

This exercise is one example of a variety of approaches that can be used to assist in managing tension, and is best used at a time of mild to moderate tension and stress. When fully developed this approach can be an important skill and resource, an activity of health.

Find a quiet place to sit and close your eyes. Feel the tension in your body. Where is it located? How does it feel? Is this your special place for feeling tension? Continue to observe the tension in your body, noticing how it fluctuates and moves from one location to the other. Your body can be an early indicator of the appearance of tension, offering you the opportunity to work with the tension before it becomes too intense. (Allow five minutes.)

Now observe your feelings, the emotions of stress. Perhaps there is anger, helplessness, frustration, sadness, or fear. There may be an initial emotion that gives way to the awareness of an underlying, more basic emotion. One sequence I often observe is: anger, fear, sadness, pain, and finally the awareness of hurt. Continue to observe the subtle shifts and changes in your emotions. You will notice that it is not a static experience, but rather one that is dynamic and changing. (Allow five minutes.)

If it is not already apparent to you, search your memory and attempt to identify the experience or interaction that shifted you into a state of tension, or perhaps even stress. Go back to the event that initiated the tension, as if it were happening right now. See the sights, hear the sounds, and feel the feelings. Allow the event to move into your body and become alive for you. If you have difficulty recalling this experience, save this exercise for another time. If not, bring the experience fully and intensely into awareness. (Allow five minutes.)

Carefully notice the setting in which this event occurred, the individuals, the space, and the time. Each element has significance. (Allow two minutes.) Work with the emotion you are experiencing, the one that seems most predominant. If it is not sufficiently intense, intensify it, turning it up as you would a faucet. Allow the feeling to take you back in time by allowing it to attach itself to earlier circumstances in your life when this same or similar feeling was present. Do not force this process; allow the emotion to do it for you, merely stating to yourself the intention to take the emotion back in time, and as you are doing this, remain focused.

Continue to go back in time to see when, where, and with whom you experienced this same feeling. Return to the earliest memory of the feeling. When the emotion attaches to a circumstance, linger for a while and observe this circumstance, seeing what you can learn from it. Continue until you have collected a "scrapbook" of these experiences. Now allow yourself to see them all in a panoramic way. What common patterns link these experiences? Did you experience helplessness, powerlessness, or victimization at another, earlier time? What resources were available for you to apply to these situations? Were the resources those of your adulthood, or childhood? Observe carefully the role you took, the role you assigned to any others, and the specific characteristics of the circumstance. You may discover a pattern that is important for you to know about. Allow the time necessary.

I would like you now to leave this place and bring yourself to a moment in your life when you were filled with confidence, competence, resourcefulness, and a sense of inner power. See it, and relive it. Be there as if it were happening in the present moment. "Turn the dial up" to make it as intense as possible, feeling it throughout your mind and body. Now, without losing this feeling, take yourself back to one or more of the previous stressful situations while holding the feeling of confidence and competence. If you lose this feeling go back to it and strengthen it before again returning to the stressful circumstance. Now relive this circumstance retaining and using these positive feelings and capacities. See what it is like when the mind changes and mature resources and capacities are brought to bear. Observe what happens to the circumstance, the other individuals, and yourself. (Allow five minutes.)

Shift back into inner silence. Do this by quietly observing your mind and/or your breathing until your mind enters silence. (Allow five minutes.) Now, from the place of silence, observe, as if you are watching a movie, all that you have done in this exercise. Do not analyze, interpret, or react to it. Merely observe it. When you are finished, slowly open your eyes and allow yourself to summarize the experience.

∽

We have used several different capacities in this exercise. First, you were able to move directly into the sources of stress as if they were happening this very moment. Next we shifted our perspectives to ones that were more positive, from those that encourage the stress response to those that assist in managing tension by conveying a sense of hardiness.

The more we know about the operations of the mind, the more we can use it to serve our purposes rather than be used by it. The more we are aware of our mental programs and how they work, the less power they have to take us over and sustain themselves. Stress, when actively engaged as an agent of health, can be a valuable teacher in life.

∾ E L E V E N ∾

HEALING IN

OUR TIME

There is hope in men, not in society, not in systems, . . . but in you and in me.

—J. Krishnamurti

Regardless of all the cultural obstacles, healing is possible because it is a personal prerogative. We cannot be healed by institutions, systems, or practices of one sort or another; we can only be healed through our own intention and our own actions. This is not the contemporary view, however. Most of us believe that healing will evolve from a reformed health-care system, better science, or alternative practices. Nothing could be further from the truth. If, for just a moment, we could look directly at the issue of healing without our preconceived notions, we would surely see that no technique, no procedure, and no organized system of beliefs can ultimately resolve our internal conflicts, conflicts that are at the source of our distress, and, not infrequently, also at the source of our ailments.

Whole Healing is not merely maintaining a steady state, or fixing and repairing with the aim of restoring normal function. Surely this is the limited aim of our Homeostatic Healing System and of the many practices, conventional and alternative, that are aspects of the treatment system. But healing is a much larger process that contains but is not defined by these approaches.

We must begin by acknowledging our current circumstance. Unable to live as we were designed to live, we resemble caged animals, locked in our limited and tenacious mental constructs. We have minds that are free, but we insist on living the biases, conceptions, and prejudices of our particular worldview—molding, shaping, and reducing the present moment to the confines of our cultural perspectives. We have intention and will, but submit ourselves to teachers, teachings, and systems of thought, right and left, that belong to others. We have the capacity to know ourselves and the world with a freshness and directness, but we satisfy ourselves with recycled projected images from our accumulated memory. We have an extraordinary built-in capacity to heal our lives, but we are satisfied with the repair and "normative" function of our physical parts.

We live relative truths, believing them to be absolute. The assumptions and principles of scientific medicine have provided us with an advanced technology and highly sophisticated diagnostic and therapeutic practices. But these very same beliefs have led to the devitalization of life and the disenchantment of nature with the all-too-apparent consequences for both individuals and the environment. Our loss of personal autonomy, the mechanization of life, unrelenting personal stress, the degradation of our natural resources, and the loss of our capacity to sustain relationship and community cannot be separated from the system of thought that has led to our technological achievements. We do not need a new worldview; we need two, ten, a thousand worldviews. Only then will we comprehend the relativeness of any system of thought and progressively learn to live without a preordained worldview. Then, no longer limited to living our preconceived notions of good and bad, primitive and advanced, healer and patient, disease and health, we will be able to dance directly with life.

In the preceding chapters I have offered a comprehensive view of our healing possibilities. I have done so not with the intention of implying that any one system can provide you with health. Nor have I offered this as an answer to particular health problems of any sort. My singular hope is that these ideas will provoke a radical reconsideration of your own thoughts and evoke a larger vision of what is possible for you and for all of us, a vision that is both uniquely personal and at the same time entirely universal.

I feel that we are blessed to have an extraordinary treatment system that is available for our use, and an increasing number of alternative therapies that we may, if we wish, choose from. I am not one who believes that all disease is "chosen" or preventable. We each age, die, and are rooted to the forces of biology. Never would I diminish the treatment resources at our disposal, or the many committed practitioners whose life's work is to assist us with these aspects of healing. But we ask too much of them—more than they can deliver. With all their wizardry and wonderful intentions they cannot perform the singular personal act of healing our lives, of preventing *premature* disease, disability, and death, and infusing joy, peace, freedom, and love into our lives.

The revolution in health and healing is not an outer one. It cannot be defined by health reform, professional organizations, insurance companies, or anyone else. These are lingering aspects of a dying singular, exclusive worldview. What we have explored is no less than a revolution in values and in perspective, a paradigm shift, or, as I have stated, hopefully one of two, ten, or a thousand paradigm shifts, a continuing shift in perspectives leaving us with a multiplicity of worldviews, a state of being that we may yet discover is the necessary antecedent of a life lived more authentically and directly. There is great hope here. I hope you see it with me.

We are living at a time of radical deconstruction of a singular, powerful worldview and the institutions and structures that have been its external manifestations. All around us we see social, political, economic, and moral decay. We are at the final phase of an important moment in the evolution of man's consciousness. From the undifferentiated consciousness of our ancestors, to the emergence of reason and inquiry in classical Greece, to the monolithic vision of the Middle Ages, and to our current era with its emphasis on a sensory-based science, an approach that allowed for a richer and more complex understanding of human life, we are at all times participants in nature's grand scheme of evolution and revelation. And because our lives are guided by the same forces that direct nature, as they become fully revealed to us, the fullness of nature is simultaneously revealed. The Christian theologian Meister Eckhart said it this way: "The eye with which God sees me is the eye through which I see him; my eye and his eye are one." Nature is articulated in human life, and human life articulates nature.

At this time in human history we have used up the value of an exclusively *objectivistic*, *deterministic*, and *positivistic* worldview. It has given us far more than we even realize. It is not only the detailed knowledge we have received, but the necessary living out of a phase in the evolution of human life, a phase that has brought us both an in-depth knowledge of certain aspects of life and the important and essential *illusion of separateness and autonomy*. It is only through this illusion that we could have learned what we have learned about human life, and, most importantly, been forced into the next phase of our development, the rediscovery of our unity with life.

To understand the necessity of the 500-year-old scientific worldview, a view that has separated mind, body, and spirit, is to understand that it was not an absurd aberration, but rather the preparation for a new worldview, one that is emerging in our time. In his book *The Passion of the Western Mind* the intellectual historian Richard Tarnas states it this way:

As the inner gestalt changes in the cultural mind, new empirical evidence just happens to appear, pertinent writings from the past are suddenly unearthed, appropriate epistemologies or justifications are formulated, supportive sociological changes coincidentally take place, new technologies become available, the telescope is invented and just happens to fall into Galileo's hands.

It is this new cultural gestalt that has given rise to the principles, assumptions, and concepts that are the essence of Whole Healing. They are not one person's image, but rather the expression of a historical movement seen through the window of health and healing. As a vehicle that will move us toward a new and more comprehensive understanding of health and healing, Whole Healing incorporates the brilliance of the scientific process but places it in a framework that is more suited to the needs and perspectives of our time.

It was 2,000 years ago that the rise of Christianity seized the creative fires from the ancient pagan gods, gods who for millennia guided humanity. A mere 500 years ago the natural sciences, in turn, seized the creative fires from Christianity, guiding the lives of our generation through the principles and values of scientific materialism. Now, in our time, when breakdown is apparent everywhere, we are finally recapturing the creative fires for *ourselves*. No longer projected outward to gods of one sort or another or encased in a rigid separatist worldview, the power for healing and self-renewal is returning home to a matured humanity capable of containing within itself the powers previously assigned first to the gods and then to science. As Charles Reich has written in *The Greening of America,*

There is a revolution coming. It will not be like revolutions of the past. It will originate in the individual and with culture and it will change the political structure only as its final act. It will not require violence to succeed and it cannot be successfully resisted with violence. It is now spreading with amazing rapidity and already our laws, in-

stitutions, and social structures are changing in consequence. It promises a higher reason, a more humane community, and a new and liberated individual. Its ultimate
creation will be a new, enduring wholeness and beauty—
a renewed relationship of man to himself, to other men,
to society, to nature, and to the land.

We have already begun to use these powers, powers that
are derived from patterns inherent in nature, to heal our lives.
As we continue, we will surely rediscover and revitalize the sacred and divine forces that throughout history have served to
guide, heal, and inspire mankind.

NOTES FROM A
FELLOW PILGRIM
SOMEWHERE ON
THE PATH

I don't know exactly what a prayer is.
I do know how to pay attention, how to fall down
into the grass, how to kneel down in the grass,
how to be idle and blessed, how to stroll through the fields,
which is what I have been doing all day.
Tell me, what else should I have done?
Doesn't everything die at last, and too soon?
Tell me, what is it you plan to do
with your one wild and precious life?

—Mary Oliver

We have now arrived at the end of our short journey together, an end that will also serve as a beginning. In the next few pages I have tried to summarize the most essential points discussed in this book. These thoughts have matured and strengthened through the many years I have explored the healing process, both in my own life and with thousands of clients. I hope you will read them, consider them, and then add your own observations.

1. *It will always be our tendency to gravitate toward treatment at the expense of broadening our vision of health.* Treatment is always easier, more efficient, and more convenient (at

least it appears that way in the short term). The current "conversation" in the alternative and complementary healing community is singularly obsessed with how to integrate alternative practices into mainstream health care and its reimbursement system. After having been a partner in over 50,000 patient visits in the 20 years of my practice (I saw each patient, one at a time, and listened carefully to their stories), I can state without question that what individuals need most in our times is "soul" work: work on their relationships, their life choices, their truncated visions and passions, and their perception of victimization and powerlessness. We need to be able to make a connection between the way we live our lives and the consequences of our choices. We need to be empowered to make change and to acknowledge an ever-present sense of the sacredness and wholeness of life. We are less in need of more professionals and practices, and more in need of a true sense of ourselves in our entirety.

2. *The healthy life is often one of estrangement from the conventional social values.* At times this can be a lonely place. Relationships are more intimate, conversations more authentic, work and play increasingly seem indistinguishable, ambition and seeking approval give way to an inner richness and self-valuing. But be prepared to be misunderstood and devalued by those who only know you by your "name" or position in life. And be similarly prepared to experience the communion that comes from those who know you beyond your name—this is where to find the true essence of intimacy and love, two profound healers.

3. *Over the many phases of a lifetime the quest for health shifts and changes.* There are specific tasks that confront us at age twenty, and others that confront us when we are thirty, forty, and so on. The idea is not to have a rigid sense of the "right" direction, but rather to listen to the moment, discern what it is asking from you, and notice in what direction life is pointing you. Every real change in life requires a deconstruction of what was, and a reconstruction of life as it must now

be. Between these two there can be long pauses of boredom, uncertainty, fear, chaos, and confusion. These are the great moments of fertility that mark the end of deconstruction and the internal preparation for a rebirth. Be patient and have faith in these periods.

4. *The aim of life is "to know one's destiny, love it, and will it."* I have previously quoted Nietzsche's famous statement from *Zarathustra*, which reflects the aspect of healing that concerns itself with discovery of personal authenticity. This means that we must let go of preconceptions, the mental constructs we have learned early in life. To know my destiny is to understand my nature, comprehend the make-up of my temperament and the character of my capacities, and discover my unique role in the universe. It is often different from what I have been taught, more than I believe, and other than I have imagined. Then I must fall in love with who I am.

When I treasure who I am, I contain and exude a self-confidence, competence, assurance, and charisma that can defy the winds of adversity and the compellingness of contemporary social values. I then use my intention and capacity to will my destiny. "How is it," you may ask, "that I will what already is destiny?" The answer is, by first not getting in the way of your natural development, and second by becoming an ally and supporter of this unfolding. To know your destiny, love it, and will it is a process that heals physiology, psychology, and spirit simultaneously.

5. *Do not be intimidated by professionals.* They do not know nearly as much as you think they do. Yes, they are quite highly educated and skilled, but their skills are narrow and only span their specialized area of interest. Time and time again I have been impressed with how much my clients know about what is occurring within their minds and bodies, and about what is needed for healing. They may not know all of the details, technical or otherwise, but they have an uncanny and often accurate sense of what needs to be done. After shar-

ing with my clients a period of meditation and silence, I often ask, "What do you feel the problem is?" I do not receive a technical answer, but that is not what I am seeking. I'm seeking a larger, intuitive sense of the full dimension of the problem. Frequently, the answers I receive astound me.

We must learn to ask our minds and bodies to reveal themselves to us, to teach us about their needs. And we must also develop the capacity to listen and to trust what we learn. After all, our minds and bodies are the storehouse of the knowledge gained through the millennia of human experience, and, at the same time, they also contain the moment-to-moment information gained through the intelligence of our homeostatic system. In many ways both these sources of knowledge surpass our cognitive knowledge in accuracy and extent. When we trust ourselves and learn from our experience, we will be able to use practitioners more effectively as the important resources they can be, rather than as the authority figures we make them out to be.

6. *Be patient with yourself.* Health and healing is a lifelong pursuit. The reward is not at the end, but rather in the day-to-day excitement that comes from new discoveries, an expanding sense of self, an ease in negotiating life, an increasing freedom from inner and outer conflict, an enhancement of inner and outer intimacies, the occasional experience of ecstasy, and the progressively more joyful awareness of the "simple" pleasures of life. The path to wholeness is not a straight line. We move between the light and dark until the dark gets filled with light, the yin and yang intermingle. As one gets accustomed to the ups and downs and the occasional return to reactive behavior, there is an increasing faith in the certainty of the process, a faith that gets stronger and stronger.

7. *Learn to love the whole of life, the gains and the losses, the sedentary moments and active ones, the good feelings and the bad feelings.* It is important for us to remember that the masks of comedy and tragedy are hung side by side. Any experience seen from one perspective assumes a different

mask when seen from another side. In one sense life is a serious endeavor, and in another sense it can be seen as an absurd joke. It is both and more. Be playful with life. The process of health and healing, irrespective of the many adversities that fuel the process, should bring joy and heartfulness to life.

8. *Until we have the strength of a fully developed consciousness we cannot at all times "hold our center."* In the *Yoga Sutras*, the ancient text by the teacher Patanjali, he advises those who are "works in progress" (a category that fits us all) on the best way to handle relationships. When we are fully developed anyone in our presence will rise in consciousness; when we are not, we are liable to find ourselves falling to the level of another. His advice is as follows: Have goodwill to those who are happy, have compassion toward those that are ill, and have benign indifference toward those that would do you harm. We must learn to choose our relationships and our environments carefully and deliberately until we become resistant to the corrosive effects of unhealthy circumstances.

9. *So much of the power of healing is bound up in the character and quality of our relationships, particularly the relationship of healer and client.* If we view ourselves as whole beings who have embodied, in the time and context of our personal lives, the mystery of existence, we must be viewed in the same way by those who share our journey toward recovery, healing, and health. That is what holism is really about. It is not, as is often thought, a technique or a practice, but rather a vision of life that *cannot* be contained or fully expressed in any one approach to treatment any more than one can package love, kindness, or spirit without limiting or distorting them. We must use our intelligence to assess the skills of a healer and our intuition to inform us that we are in a rich, non-judgmental, intimate, and acknowledging communion. We make too much of treatments, conventional and alternative, and not enough of the quality of relationship through which we receive them. This was not so in earlier times, when the lack of technology allowed time and concern for the more

personal aspects of healing. It is unnecessary to give up technology to recapture the wonderful elixir of healing that is woven into the tapestry of healing relationships.

10. *Remember that compassion heals both healer and client.* The term *compassion* is a particularly important word in the Buddhist tradition. Compassion is the capacity to experience directly the circumstance of another. It is not a cognitive understanding, but more an empathic communion. It is born from the wisdom that comprehends that our individual journeys are merely multiple expressions of a singular shared journey, and from the knowledge that arises from living through the experience of pain and suffering. Compassion brings me into a direct intimacy with life by breaking down the surface distinctions that separate you from me. It is a surrender to the larger forces of life of which we are all a part. It both humbles me and makes me larger.

Our lives are given to us as unformed potential. From the undeveloped possibilities of the infant to the still unfolding possibilities of a conscious adult, we are always in a dynamic state of being and becoming. These possibilities can be shaped and limited from the outside, as they often are, or evolve from the inside. In the first instance we have little involvement and surrender our essential humanity to the forces of culture (of which treatment is one); in the second instance we orchestrate our own lives and in this manner most fully live out our healing potential and our destiny. In this choice lies all of the difference.

Bibliography

Recommending books, periodicals or organizations has never been easy for me. My approach is only to recommend what I have personally experienced and know to be of value. The listings in this appendix are not complete. There are many other resources that are of value. This is, however, a good place to begin.

Chapter One: Whole Healing

The major sources for the ideas expressed in *Whole Healing* can be found in the work of George Engel, which is predominantly described in a series of journal articles, and von Bertalanffy's exposition of systems theory as referenced below.

Engel, George, "The Clinical Application of the Biopsychosocial Model," *The American Journal of Psychiatry* (1980:137), pp. 535–544.

———, "A Unified Concept of Health and Disease," *Perspectives in Biology and Medicine* (Summer 1960), pp. 459–485.

————, "The Need for a New Medical Model: A Challenge for Bio-medicine," *Science* (1977:196), pp. 129–136.

CHAPTER TWO: THE CENTRE CANNOT HOLD

Kuhn, T. S., *The Structure of Scientific Revolutions*. Chicago: University of Chicago Press, 1970.

Von Bertalanffy, L., *General Systems Theory*. New York: Braziller, 1968.

Systems theory is a science of wholeness. This book, which is at times erudite, takes us through a step-by-step understanding of systems theory and its application to our lives. I have found it quite difficult to shift my patterned ways and begin to see wholes rather than parts; this book has helped the process of reshaping how I approach life. An in-depth understanding of Whole Healing is assisted by an understanding of systems theory.

Weiss, P., "The System of Nature and the Nature of Systems: Empirical Holism and Practical Reductionism Harmonized," in *Toward a Man-Centered Science*, edited by Schaeffer, K. E., Hensel H., Brody, R. Mount Kisco, N.Y.: Futura, 1977.

In 1975 a small group of physicians, philosophers, social scientists, and medical administrators met, under the auspices of the Rocke-feller Foundation, to explore ideas about health and the delivery of health care. This is one of a series of essays that emerged from this meeting. It demonstrates the application of systems theory to biology, and our ideas about health. It is highly recommended.

CHAPTER THREE: THE HOMEOSTATIC HEALING SYSTEM

Locke, Stephen, *The Healer Within*. New York: E. P. Dutton, 1986.

Dr. Locke, a prominent investigator in the field of PNI, provides us with an informed overview of the developing understanding of the mind/body interaction. This is a good, basic, readable introduction to the field.

Cannon, W. B., *The Wisdom of the Body*. New York: W. W. Norton, 1931.

This classic book establishes the early scientific foundation for the homeostatic system. Although the content is now dated, as with all great thinkers Cannon provides us with timeless insights and understandings into our primary self-healing system.

CHAPTER FOUR: THE TREATMENT HEALING SYSTEM

A Report to the National Institutes of Health, *Alternative Medicine: Expanding Medical Horizons*. U.S. Superintendent of Documents, P.O. Box 371954, Pittsburgh, PA. 15250; Document # 7578.

This report was prepared under the auspices of a workshop on alternative medicine held in 1992 and supported by the Office of Alternative Medicine of the National Institutes of Health. The report reviews the current status of multiple treatment modalities, issues regarding research, and an appendix that supports and expands upon this work. This is a valuable tool for gathering additional information on treatment approaches.

Illich, Ivan, *Medical Nemesis*. New York: Pantheon, 1976.

Having first read this book at publication time, I recently reread it and marveled at Illich's observations. However extreme his conclusions may at times seem, there can be little doubt that the essence of his observations regarding the overt and covert effects of biomedicine are timely, accurate, and deeply disturbing. This is a "must read" book.

CHAPTER FIVE: CONSCIOUSNESS: THE ACTIVATING FACTOR

Goldstein, J., *The Experience of Insight*. Boulder, Colo.: Shambala, 1987.

This important book is a detailed introduction to the practice of mindfulness. It is clear, concise, and greatly expands upon the information in this chapter.

Goldstein, J., and Kornfield, J., *Seeking the Heart of Wisdom*. Boston and London: Shambala, 1987.

This is a companion book to *The Experience of Insight*. Well written and highly recommended, it expands upon the previously presented concepts, drawing the reader into an increasingly deeper understanding of mindfulness.

Krishnamurti, J., *Freedom from the Known*. New York: Harper & Row, 1969.

One reads Krishnamurti to experience his extraordinary analysis of the problems of modern times, and his precise, brilliant, and mindful intelligence. In this book he explores the issue of personal freedom, which he believes develops as we shift from a conditioned mind that lives in the past to a creative mind that lives in the here and now. It is an excellent complement to the other readings on insight and mindfulness.

Kornfield, J., and Breiter, Paul, *A Still Forest Pool: The Insight Meditation of Achaan Chah*. Wheaton, Ill.: Theosophical Publishing House, 1985.

This wonderful, sweet book introduces the reader to the wisdom of mindfulness as expressed by a skilled teacher and wise man. The writing is clear, the little parables wonderful, and in time you begin to assimilate the feeling and teachings of the monastic life, much of which is applicable to modern-day living.

Bridges, William, *Transitions*. Reading, Mass.: Addison-Wesley, 1980.

As we undertake the journey toward health and wholeness, it is valuable to take a blueprint with you. Bridges provides such a blueprint in this book. It is a thoughtful and heartfelt exploration of the stages of transition, a process, I have concluded, that once started, lasts a lifetime.

Thoreau, H. D., *Walden*. New York: Doubleday, 1954.

This wonderful classic provides us with Thoreau's reflections on self and life in the solitude of Walden Pond. It is one man's primer on silence and observer/inquiring consciousness.

CHAPTER SIX: THE MIND/BODY HEALING SYSTEM

Dacher, E., *Intentional Healing*. New York: Marlowe, 1996.

Goleman, Daniel, and Gurin, Joel, *Mind/Body Medicine*. New York: Consumer Reports Books, 1993.

In my view, this is the most comprehensive, thoughtful, and re-sourceful exposition of the issues of mind/body healing that is currently available in print. This book, a compendium of articles contributed by well-regarded teachers and clinicians, covers theory and practice. It is full of well-annotated references and resources.

Swami Hariharananda Aranya, *The Yoga Philosophy of Patanjali*. Albany: State University of New York Press, 1983.

This book is not for everyone. It requires much time with each word, sentence, and paragraph, as well as considerable patience with a new vocabulary. The reward is equal to the effort. This book, commonly referred to as the *Yoga Sutras*, is a complete science of the mind. It is a detailed description of how the mind works, and how to work with it.

Green, Elmer and Alyce, *Beyond Biofeedback*. New York: Delta, 1977.

This wonderful, readable, and wise book, written by the pioneers of biofeedback and self-regulation, is filled with research data, personal experiences, and clinical observations. The authors re-view topics such as homeostasis, self-regulation, biofeedback training, the role of biofeedback in the treatment of specific disor-ders, body consciousness, mind training, and volition.

Yalom, Irving, *When Nietzsche Wept*. New York: Basic Books, 1992.

A wonderful exploration of the beginnings of our modern-day approach to expanding consciousness, the "talking cure," otherwise know as psychotherapy. This novel explores the fictional meeting of Joseph Breuer and Friedrich Nietzsche through which they explore the nature of self and existence, concurrently healing each other's despair.

Storr, Anthony, *Solitude, A Return to the Self*. New York: Free Press, 1988.

Although a bit erudite, this book examines an important and infrequently discussed issue. Contrary to the perspectives of Western society, which often measures well-being by the capacity to succeed in relationships, Storr makes the case that true health and happiness result from the capacity to live at peace with oneself. He explores the relationships of solitude to creativity, self-growth, healing, and the religious experience.

The Portable Jung. Edited by Joseph Campbell, New York: Penguin, 1971.

This is a selection of the most accessible works of Jung. I would particularly recommend the readings in Part I, and the first and last two readings in Part II. In my view, Jung thoroughly understood the process of human development and the expansion of consciousness that lead toward health and wholeness. This book is worth the time it will take you, and perhaps it is important to move through it slowly.

Joy, Brugh, *Avalanche*. New York: Ballantine, 1990.

Brugh Joy is a physician who left his practice many years ago to explore an expanded and multidimensional approach to healing. Unlike many others, he has been willing to engage the darker aspect of life as a vehicle toward a healthier and more conscious existence. *Avalanche* is his most recent exploration of his journey into the psyche and discovery of its vast resources.

Pilusk, Marc, and Parks, Susan, H., *The Healing Web: Social Networks and Human Survival.* Hanover, N.H.: University Press of New England, 1986.

This book is the place to start if you wish to pursue further the field of social support and its relationship to health and healing.

Kabat-Zinn, Jon, *Full Catastrophe Living.* New York: Delta, 1990.

In this book, Dr. Kabat-Zinn reports on his multiyear experience with his Stress Reduction and Relaxation Program for individuals suffering from physical or emotional distress. This book is well done and provides the reader with significant insight into the sources of stress and the practical solutions that work at the sources.

Johnson, R., *We.* Cambridge, Mass.: Harper & Row, 1983.

This marvelous short book explores the Western notion of romance. It examines the relationship of romance to the practical and spiritual aspects of life. Through the classical story of Tristan and Isolde, he suggests answers to our recurring questions about the role of intimate relationships in our lives.

Fromm, Eric, *The Art of Loving.* New York: Harper & Row, 1956.

In this classic work, the author, in a concise, simple, and wise manner, discusses the nature of love and provides a practical set of guidelines that may assist individuals in creating healthy loving relationships.

Pelletier, Kenneth R., *Mind as Healer, Mind as Slayer.* New York: Peter Smith, 1984.

Although years old, this book remains one of the best explorations of the nature and meaning of stress. As the title suggests, it is a good companion to *Whole Healing.*

CHAPTER SEVEN: THE SPIRITUAL HEALING SYSTEM

Daumal, Rene, *Mount Analogue*. Boston: Shambala, 1986.

One of my favorites. Mountains are metaphors for the connection between the earth and the heavens. In this marvelous story, Daumal teaches us about the journey to wholeness: the ascent, the plateaus, the obstacles, the challenges, and the rewards. It is short, concise, and beautifully written.

Jung, C. G., *Mysterium Coniunctionis*. Princeton, N.J.: Princeton University Press, 1963.

This book is not for everyone. It is very difficult reading. Yet it provides the reader with an extraordinary scholarly understanding of the nature of wholeness, and its step-by-step achievement through the process of human development. I have used this text as a major source for Chapters 6 and 7.

Berry, Thomas, *The Dream of the Earth*. San Francisco: Sierra Club Books, 1988.

This wonderful and scholarly book makes a compelling case for the earth. Many important facts and issues are presented. The author, urging us to consider ourselves as a vanguard of the next era, the ecological era, describes a step-by-step approach to global healing. This is an important book to read.

Whitman, Walt, *Leaves of Grass*. New York: Doubleday, 1960.

In this American classic, Whitman demonstrates an extraordinary capacity for mindfulness. Whitman's observations of the experiences of daily life are inspiring examples of how to live a mindful life.

CHAPTER EIGHT: CLOSE ONE DOOR AND OPEN ANOTHER

Antonovsky, Aaron, *Health, Stress, and Coping.* San Francisco: Jossey-Bass, 1969.

Antonovsky, Aaron, *Unraveling the Mystery of Health.* San Francisco: Jossey-Bass, 1987.

In these two books, Antonovsky proposes a proactive vision of health. He views health as the development of specific personal qualities, which, when taken together, afford an ongoing resistance to stress-induced disease.

Pietroni, Patrick, *The Greening of Medicine.* London: Victor Gollancz, 1990.

This superb book traces the history of the development of scientific medicine, explores its problems, and looks toward future solutions. I found this book an easy-to-read, highly informative, and thoughtful exploration of the issues posed by our current approaches to medical care.

Dossey, Larry, *Meaning and Medicine.* New York: Bantam, 1991.

Dossey, from the perspective of a practicing physician, offers the reader a new vision of health and healing, one that clearly fits with what we have discussed in this book. He covers the territory of mind/body healing, but, much to our advantage, seems most at home in his exploration of spiritual healing.

Choiceless Awareness, A Selection of Passages for the Study of the Teachings of J. Krishnamurti, Krishnamurti Foundation of America (see resource section for full address).

A wonderful collection of the writings of Krishnamurti that outline the general principles of the new way of thinking discussed in Chapter 9.

Storr, Paul, *The Social Transformation of American Medicine.* New York: Basic Books, 1982.

This scholarly book traces the development of American medicine, as a profession and industry, from the mid-eighteenth century to the present date. It discusses the successes, failures, and future directions of our medical care system. If you have a special interest in a more detailed understanding of these issues, this book can serve as a good resource.

Needleman, J., *The Way of the Physician.* San Francisco: Harper & Row, 1985.

The author examines the predicaments, ideals, and challenges of modern medicine and the physicians who practice it. He looks toward the future and explores how we can recapture the ideals and humanism of medicine. It is wonderful reading filled with personal recollections, up-to-date knowledge, and the wisdom of this philosopher.

CHAPTER NINE: THE QUALITIES OF HEALTH

Important reading for this chapter includes Aaron Antonovsky (see Chapter 1 and Chapter 8), Erik Erikson (see Chapter 3), and Suzanne Kobassa (see Chapter 7).

Maslow, Abraham, *Motivation and Personality.* New York: Harper and Row, 1954.

Maslow's work in exploring and delineating the field of developmental psychology is very central to the efforts in this book. His chapter on self-actualizing people is highly thoughtful, and in my view, it is still one of the best available resources as regards the full spectrum of qualities found in healthy people.

Rogers, Carl, *On Becoming a Person.* Boston: Houghton Mifflin, 1961.

As with the other pioneers in the field of developmental psychology, Rogers developed a keen interest in the qualities and characteristics of the healthy individual. In this book, he provides us with his thoughtful views on this issue as well as reviewing some other fundamental considerations.

CHAPTER ELEVEN: HEALING IN OUR TIME

Richard Tarnas, *The Passion of the Western Mind.* New York: Ballantine, 1991.

In this exceptional book Tarnas weaves the threads of Western thought from Plato and Aristotle to Jung. Through his capacity to synthesize and intuit patterns and relationships, he provides us with an important historical context that informs us about the sources and directions of the shifts and changes emerging in our times. As usual, proper understanding underlies proper action.

༄

PERIODICALS

Advances. The Fetzer Institute, 9292 West KL Avenue, Kalamazoo, Michigan 49009.

The goal of this quarterly publication, and occasional supplemental mailings, is "the expansion and communication of knowledge about the integration of mind and body in health and disease." The articles, book reviews, and calendar of events are good sources of information for individuals who wish a continuous update on current issues in mine/body healing.

Alternative Therapies in Health and Medicine. 101 Columbia Avenue, Aliso Viejo, California 92656.

The Journal of Alternative and Complementary Medicine: Research on Practice, Paradigm, and Policy. Mary Ann Liebert, Inc. 1651 Third Avenue, New York, New York 10128.

The above two journals are recent additions to the available literature in alternative and complementary medicine. I recommend them both.

Berkeley Wellness Letter. University of California, P.O. Box 42014, Palm Coast, Florida 32142.

This monthly newsletter offers its readers a variety of articles on nutrition, fitness, and stress management. Its focus is on prevention.

Nutrition Action. Center for Science in the Public Interest, 1501 Sixteenth Street, N.W., Washington, D.C. 20077.

This is the best up-to-date, reliable, well-presented source of nutrition information I have found. The monthly magazine and the variety of valuable posters and booklets provide the subscriber with a comprehensive set of resources.

Parabola. The Society of Myth and Tradition, 656 Broadway, New York, New York 10012.

This beautiful, informative, and highly inspirational magazine explores a different topic each quarter. Contributing writers offer their comments on topics such as wholeness, the hero, disciples and discipline, addiction, forgiveness, and many others.

Resources

The Institute of Noetic Sciences, 475 Gate Five Road, Suite #300, Sausalito, California 94965.

IONS, through its quarterly review and publications, is an ongoing source of information regarding healing and consciousness.

The Krishnamurti Foundation of America, P.O. Box 1560, Ojai, California 93024.

This organization continues the work of Krishnamurti. They offer a variety of programs, retreats, and educational materials related to mindfulness and self-healing.

Esalen Institute, Big Sur, California 93920.

The Omega Institute, Lake Drive R.D. 2, Box 377, Rhinebeck, New York 12572.

The Kripalu Center, P.O. Box 793, Lenox, Massachusetts 01240.

The New York Open Center, 83 Spring Street, New York, New York 10012.

Interface, 522 Main Street, Watertown, Massachusetts 02172.

Each of these centers provides a variety of programs dealing with issues such as meditation, health and healing, movement, personal development, Yoga, and environmental and global issues.

The Fetzer Institute, 9292 West KL Avenue, Kalamazoo, Michigan 49009.

The work and publications of the Fetzer Institute, the publisher of *Advances* and the prime contributor to the Bill Moyers *Healing and the Mind* series, is an important resource for all those interested in mind/body healing.

Insight Meditation Society, Pleasant Street, Barre, Massachusetts 01001.

Insight Meditation West, P.O. Box 909, Woodacre, California 94973.

Both these organizations offer three-, ten-, thirty-, and ninety-day intensive mindfulness meditation retreats. These retreats are an opportunity for intensive study under the guidance of skilled teachers. They are highly recommended for both beginners and advanced students.

Commonweal, P.O. Box 316, Bolinas, California 94924.

This is an education and training center that assists individuals with cancer in exploring complementary forms of healing that will enable the individual to work more effectively with cancer to maximize self-healing and "expand" life. This program is highly recommended. Available through Commonweal is a well-written, well-researched, and thoughtful compendium on alternative approaches to cancer.

FOR FURTHER INFORMATION

If you would like further information on workshops, seminars, publications, and other materials related to Whole Healing, we would welcome hearing from you. Please write to us at:

Whole Healing
Gay Head, Massachusetts 02535

INDEX

· A NOTE ON THE TYPE ·

The typeface used in this book is a version of Century (Expanded), originally designed by Theodore L. De Vinne (1828–1914) and Linn Boyd Benton for De Vinne's *Century* magazine; it was probably the first type developed for such a specific purpose. De Vinne, an innovative though practical printer and a scholar of typography, thought the type then used in periodicals feeble and proposed that the thin strokes of the "modern" typefaces be thickened while keeping the economical narrow letter forms so characteristic of late-nineteenth-century fonts (one of the "ungenerous" aspects of contemporary type that made William Morris look to the past). Century was later developed for wider use by Benton's son, Morris Fuller Benton (1872–1948), who did more than anyone else to advance the concept of a type "family"—several "weights" of a typeface with uniform design.